Sedation and Monitoring in Gastrointestinal Endoscopy

Editor

JOHN J. VARGO

GASTROINTESTINAL ENDOSCOPY CLINICS OF NORTH AMERICA

www.giendo.theclinics.com

Consulting Editor
CHARLES J. LIGHTDALE

July 2016 • Volume 26 • Number 3

ELSEVIER

1600 John F. Kennedy Boulevard • Suite 1800 • Philadelphia, Pennsylvania, 19103-2899

http://www.theclinics.com

GASTROINTESTINAL ENDOSCOPY CLINICS OF NORTH AMERICA Volume 26, Number 3
July 2016 ISSN 1052-5157, ISBN-13: 978-0-323-44845-1

Editor: Kerry Holland
Developmental Editor: Donald Mumford

Gastrointestinal Endoscopy Clinics of North America (ISSN 1052-5157) is published quarterly by Elsevier Inc., 360 Park Avenue South, New York, NY 10010-1710. Months of issue are January, April, July, and October. Business and Editorial Offices: 1600 John F. Kennedy Blvd., Suite 1800, Philadelphia, PA, 19103-2899. Periodicals postage paid at New York, NY and additional mailing offices. Subscription prices are $335.00 per year for US individuals, $538.00 per year for US institutions, $100.00 per year for US students and residents, $370.00 per year for Canadian individuals, $637.00 per year for Canadian institutions, $465.00 per year for international individuals, $637.00 per year for international institutions, and $245.00 per year for Canadian and foreign students/residents. To receive student/resident rate, orders must be accompanied by name of affiliated institution, date of term, and the *signature* of program/residency coordinator on institution letterhead. Orders will be billed at individual rate until proof of status is received. Foreign air speed delivery is included in all *Clinics* subscription prices. All prices are subject to change without notice. **POSTMASTER:** Send address change to *Gastrointestinal Endoscopy Clinics of North America*, Elsevier Health Sciences Division, Subscription Customer Service, 3251 Riverport Lane, Maryland Heights, MO 63043. **Customer Service: 1-800-654-2452 (US). From outside the United States, call 1-314-447-8871. Fax: 1-314-447-8029. E-mail: JournalsCustomerService-usa@elsevier.com (for print support) or JournalsOnlineSupport-usa@elsevier.com (for online support).**

Reprints. For copies of 100 or more, of articles in this publication, please contact the Commercial Reprints Department, Elsevier Inc., 360 Park Avenue South, New York, NY 10010-1710. Tel. 212-633-3874; Fax: 212-633-3820; E-mail: reprints@elsevier.com.

Gastrointestinal Endoscopy Clinics of North America is covered in *Excerpta Medica, MEDLINE/PubMed (Index Medicus), and MEDLINE/MEDLARS.*

Contributors

CONSULTING EDITOR

CHARLES J. LIGHTDALE, MD
Professor of Medicine, Division of Digestive and Liver Diseases, Columbia University Medical Center, New York, New York

EDITOR

JOHN J. VARGO, MD, MPH, AGAF, FACP, FACG, FASGE
Chairman, Department of Gastroenterology and Hepatology, Pier C. and Renee A. Borra Family Endowed Chair in Gastroenterology and Hepatology; Vice Chairman, Digestive Disease and Surgery Institute, Cleveland Clinic, Cleveland Clinic Foundation, Cleveland, Ohio

AUTHORS

TYLER M. BERZIN, MD, MS
Associate Professor of Medicine, Center for Advanced Endoscopy, Beth Israel Deaconess Medical Center, Harvard Medical School, Boston, Massachusetts

SEKAR BHAVANI, MD, MS, FRCS (I)
Institute of Anesthesiology, Staff Anesthesiologist; Section Head for NORA; Associate Program Director; Assistant Professor, CCLCM, Cleveland Clinic, Cleveland, Ohio

JAMES BUXBAUM, MD
Director of Endoscopy, Los Angeles Couty Hospital, Division of Gastroenterology and Liver Diseases, Keck School of Medicine, University of Southern California, Los Angeles, California

HYUN KEE CHUNG, MD
Chief, Pediatric Anesthesia, Department of Anesthesia, UMass Memorial Medical Center; Associate Professor of Anesthesiology, University of Massachusetts Medical School, Worcester, Massachusetts

BEN DA, MD
Division of Gastroenterology and Liver Diseases, Keck School of Medicine, University of Southern California, Los Angeles, California

ANDREW D. FELD, MD, JD
Program Chief, Group Health Cooperative; Clinical Professor of Medicine, University of Washington, Seattle, Washington

KAYLA A. FELD, JD
University of Washington, Seattle, Washington

ANANT GILL, MBBS
Saraswathi Institute of Medical Sciences, Anwarpur, Uttar Pradesh, India

ZACHARY P. HARRIS, MD
Department of Medicine, University of Arkansas for Medical Sciences, Little Rock, Arkansas

PICHAMOL JIRAPINYO, MD
Gastroenterology Fellow, Division of Gastroenterology, Hepatology and Endoscopy, Brigham and Women's Hospital, Harvard Medical School, Boston, Massachusetts

GURSIMRAN S. KOCHHAR, MD, FACP
Department of Gastroenterology and Hepatology, Digestive Disease and Surgery Institute, Cleveland Clinic, Cleveland, Ohio

ANDREAS A. KRALIOS, JD
University of Washington, Seattle, Washington

JENIFER R. LIGHTDALE, MD, MPH
Division Chief, Pediatric Gastroenterology and Nutrition, UMass Memorial Children's Medical Center; Professor of Pediatrics, University of Massachusetts Medical School, Worcester, Massachusetts

JULIA LIU, MD, MSc, FACG, FACP, FASGE
Department of Medicine, University of Arkansas for Medical Sciences, Little Rock, Arkansas

NADIM MAHMUD, MD, MS, MPH
Instructor of Medicine, Department of Internal Medicine, Brigham and Women's Hospital, Harvard Medical School, Boston, Massachusetts

WALTER G. MAURER, MD
Staff, Department of General Anesthesia, Cleveland Clinic, Cleveland, Ohio

PAUL NIKLEWSKI, PhD
Department of Pharmacology and Cell Biophysics, University of Cincinnati College of Medicine; Xavier University; Sedasys, a Division of Ethicon Endo-Surgery, Inc, Cincinnati, Ohio

DANIEL PAMBIANCO, MD
Charlottesville Medical Research, Charlottesville, Virginia

DOUGLAS K. REX, MD, MACP, MACG, FASGE, AGAF
Distinguished Professor of Medicine, Indiana University School of Medicine; Director of Endoscopy, Indiana University Hospital, Indianapolis, Indiana

JOHN R. SALTZMAN, MD, FACP, FACG, FASGE, AGAF
Director of Endoscopy, Brigham and Women's Hospital; Associate Professor of Medicine, Harvard Medical School, Boston, Massachusetts

JOHN E. TETZLAFF, MD
Professor of Anesthesiology; Cleveland Clinic Lerner College of Medicine of Case Western Reserve University Staff, Department of General Anesthesia, Cleveland Clinic, Cleveland, Ohio

CHRISTOPHER C. THOMPSON, MD, MSc, FACG, FASGE
Director of Therapeutic Endoscopy, Division of Gastroenterology, Hepatology and Endoscopy, Brigham and Women's Hospital, Associate Professor of Medicine, Harvard Medical School, Boston, Massachusetts

JOHN J. VARGO, MD, MPH, AGAF, FACP, FACG, FASGE
Chairman, Department of Gastroenterology and Hepatology, Pier C. and Renee A. Borra Family Endowed Chair in Gastroenterology and Hepatology; Vice Chairman, Digestive Disease Institute, Cleveland Clinic, Cleveland Clinic Foundation, Cleveland, Ohio

JOSEPH J. VICARI, MD
Rockford Gastroenterology Associates, Ltd; Department of Medicine, University of Illinois College of Medicine at Rockford, Rockford, Illinois

Contents

The role of the anesthesia service in sedation for gastrointestinal endoscopy (GIE) has been steadily increasing. The goals of preprocedural assessment are determined by the specific details of the procedure, the issues related to the illness that requires the endoscopy, comorbidities, the goals for sedation, and the risk of complications from the sedation and the endoscopic procedure. Rather than consider these issues as separate entities, they should be considered as part of a continuum of preparation for GIE. This is told from the perspective of an anesthesiologist who regularly participates in the full range of sedation for GIE.

The practice of endoscopic sedation requires a thorough understanding of preprocedural assessment, sedation pharmacology, intraprocedure monitoring, adverse event management, and postprocedural care. The training process has become increasingly standardized and entails knowledge and practice-based components. The use of propofol in particular requires a higher level of structured training owing to its narrow therapeutic window. Simulation has increased opportunities for practice-based training in a controlled environment. After completion of training, the endoscopist must demonstrate competence in theoretical understanding and technical ability to administer sedation. Although individual institutions have certification processes, there is a lack of validated, standardized methods to confirm competence.

Goals of endoscopic sedation are to provide patients with a successful procedure, and ensure that they remain safe and are relieved from anxiety and discomfort; agents should provide efficient, appropriate sedation and allow patients to recover rapidly. Sedation is usually safe and effective; however, complications may ensue. This paper outlines some medicolegal aspects of endoscopic sedation, including informed consent, possible withdrawal of consent during the procedure, standard of care for monitoring sedation, use of anesthesia personnel to deliver sedation, and new agents and devices.

Sekar Bhavani

The term, *non–operating room anesthesia*, describes a location remote from the main operating suites and closer to the patient, including areas that offer specialized procedures, like endoscopy suites, cardiac catheterization laboratories, bronchoscopy suites, and invasive radiology suites. There has been an exponential growth in such procedures and they present challenges in both organizational aspects and administration of anesthesia. This article explores the requirements for the location, preoperative evaluation and patient selection, monitoring, anesthesia technique, and postoperative management at these sites. There is a need to better define the role of the anesthesia personnel at these remote sites.

Douglas K. Rex

Endoscopist-directed propofol (EDP) refers to delivery of propofol for endoscopic sedation under the direction of an endoscopist without any involvement of an anesthesia specialist (anesthesiologist or nurse anesthetist). EDP has been proven to be safe and is also cost-effective compared with the anesthetist delivered sedation for endoscopy. EDP has been endorsed by US gastroenterology societies as an appropriate paradigm for clinical practice. EDP has proliferated in Switzerland and Germany, but its expansion in the United States has been limited by financial disincentives, concerns about medical-legal risk for endoscopists, and regulatory obstacles.

Nadim Mahmud and Tyler M. Berzin

Gastrointestinal endoscopic sedation has improved procedural and patient outcomes but is associated with attendant risks of oversedation and hemodynamic compromise. Therefore, close monitoring during endoscopic procedures using sedation is critical. This monitoring begins with appropriate staff trained in visual assessment of patients and analysis of basic physiologic parameters. It also mandates an array of devices widely used in practice to evaluate hemodynamics, oxygenation, ventilation, and depth of sedation. The authors review the evidence behind monitoring practices and current society recommendations and discuss forthcoming technologies and techniques that are poised to improve noninvasive monitoring of patients under endoscopic sedation.

Hyun Kee Chung and Jenifer R. Lightdale

Sedation is a fundamental component of pediatric gastrointestinal procedures. The 2 main types of sedation for pediatric endoscopy remain general anesthesia and procedural sedation. Although anesthesiologist-administered sedation protocols are more common, there is no ideal regimen for endoscopy in children. This article discusses specific levels of sedation for endoscopy as well as various regimens that can be used to achieve each. Risks and considerations that may be specific to performing gastrointestinal procedures in children are reviewed. Finally, potential future directions for sedation and monitoring that may change the practice of pediatric gastroenterology and ultimately patient outcomes are examined.

This article reviews the data for diagnostic and uncomplicated therapeutic upper endoscopy, which show it is safe and effective to perform the procedure under moderate sedation with a combination of benzodiazepine and opioids. For more complex procedures or for superobese patients anesthesia support is recommended. Performing endoscopy in this population should alert providers to plan carefully and individualize sedation plans because there is no objective way to quantify this risk pre-endoscopically.

In the United States, sedation and analgesia are the standard of practice when endoscopic procedures are performed in the ambulatory endoscopy center. Over the last 30 years, there has been a dramatic shift of endoscopic procedures from the hospital outpatient department to ambulatory endoscopy centers. This article will discuss sedation and analgesia in the ambulatory endoscopy center as it relates to optimizing safety, patient expectations, and efficiency.

Recent development and expansion of endoscopy units has necessitated similar progress in the quality assurance of procedure sedation and monitoring. The large number of endoscopic procedures performed annually underlies the need for standardized quality initiatives focused on mitigating patient risk before, during, and immediately after endoscopic sedation, as well as improving procedure outcomes and patient satisfaction. Specific standards are needed for newer sedation modalities, including propofol administration. This article reviews the current guidelines and literature concerning quality assurance and endoscopic procedure sedation.

As the number and complexity of endoscopic procedures increase, the role of sedation has been integral in patient and physician satisfaction. This article discusses the advances of computer-assisted and patient-controlled platforms. These computer-assisted and patient-controlled platforms use different anesthetics and analgesics, all with the intent of achieving improved consistency in the level of sedation, appropriate to the needs of patients, while also improving patient safety. These systems have been around for decades; however, few are approved for use in the United States, and several still require further study before broad clinical application.

On the Horizon: The Future of Procedural Sedation   577

Gursimran S. Kochhar, Anant Gill, and John J. Vargo

Sedation plays an integral part in endoscopy. By achieving patient comfort, it allows for a better examination and enhances patient satisfaction. Various medications have been used, propofol being the current favorite. With emphasis on patient safety and quality of endoscopy, various new medications in different combinations are being used to achieve adequate sedation and not escalate the cost of the procedure. With the advent of newer medications and newer modalities to administer these medications, there is need for more specialized training for the endoscopist to feel comfortable while using these medications.

GASTROINTESTINAL ENDOSCOPY CLINICS OF NORTH AMERICA

THE CLINICS ARE AVAILABLE ONLINE!
Access your subscription at:
www.theclinics.com

Foreword

Sedation for Gastrointestinal Endoscopy: An Uneasy State of the Art

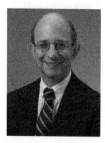

Charles J. Lightdale, MD
Consulting Editor

Ask any endoscopist to dream of an ideal sedation regimen for gastrointestinal endoscopy, and we all give the same description. It would have a quick onset, be very effective in everyone, be very safe, and result in rapid recovery with happy patients walking out the door. Oh, and it should be administered under the control of the gastrointestinal endoscopist. Unfortunately, to be honest, endoscopists have never had anything close to this ideal.

For as long as we have performed endoscopy, we have always needed sedation for most cases in order to provide patient comfort and a quiet field to carry out successful examination or therapy. Historically, our first regimens relied on opioids and barbiturates, which were clunky to use and variably effective. The benzodiazepines then became the norm, and combinations of midazolam and fentanyl became popular. Many of us may still remember in the 1990s when the virtues of this regimen were extolled. As endoscopists, we marveled at its ability to work within 5 to 10 minutes, while being admonished to administer each drug in small increments. Alas, while benzodiazepines and opioids remain sufficient for most patients, it is also clear that they don't work for a significant minority, including some who experience agitation, insufficient sedation, or excessive sedation. Recovery times can be very long and can be associated with long hangover symptoms.

The not-so-newest agent on the block, propofol, offers some definite benefits. When we all first starting using it about 20 years ago, the opaque white liquid was jokingly dubbed "the milk of amnesia." It is extremely rapid-acting and puts practically everybody to sleep within a minute. Propofol is also cleared relatively quickly and has a fast recovery, helping unit efficiency and easing pressure on recovery space. However, its therapeutic window is narrow. Respiratory depression can occur with remarkable speed, and there are no agents to reverse its effects, unlike the case for opioids and

Gastrointest Endoscopy Clin N Am 26 (2016) xiii–xiv
http://dx.doi.org/10.1016/j.giec.2016.04.001
1052-5157/16/$ – see front matter © 2016 Published by Elsevier Inc.

benzodiazepines. Patients with obesity and sleep apnea syndromes receiving propofol are particularly prone to developing obstructive airway problems.

Still, as we have worked with it, large amounts of data have accumulated, which have indicated that gastrointestinal endoscopists can use propofol as safely as combinations of opioids and benzodiazepines. However, in the United States, endoscopist-administered propofol has been forced to cease under unwavering pressure from anesthesiology societies, who have convinced numerous federal and state regulatory agencies to restrict the use of propofol to certified anesthesia specialists.

Therefore, the current use of sedation and monitoring for gastrointestinal endoscopy in the United States involves either endoscopist-administered sedation using opioids and benzodiazepines, or anesthesiologist-administered sedation using propofol. Many high-throughput endoscopy centers are using anesthesiologist-administered propofol exclusively for sedation. Hospital-based endoscopists doing complex, lengthy, therapeutic procedures also have become high users of anesthesiologist-administered propofol.

There is no doubt that considerable authority and control in many gastrointestinal endoscopy units have been ceded to anesthesiology. Many endoscopists currently start a procedure day knowing it will be dictated by their assigned anesthesiologist or supervised nurse-anesthetist. Yet, while anesthesia specialists generally speaking have more experience rescuing patients from sedation-related respiratory depression than endoscopists, anesthesiologists and nurse anesthetists are certainly not always perfect or free from complications. Instead, there are remarkably different ways that propofol is administered by anesthesia specialists, often with mixed results. In the absence of fixed protocols for propofol administration for gastrointestinal procedures, it has become evident that some anesthesia specialists are more skilled at it than others. Costs for anesthesiology services for gastrointestinal endoscopy have escalated, while reimbursements for gastrointestinal endoscopists have been reduced. How this will all play out in the long transition from fee-for-service to global value-based reimbursement for our procedures remains an open question.

It seemed clear to me that we needed an issue of the *Gastrointestinal Endoscopy Clinics of North America* that would help us navigate this new and uneasy state-of-the-art of sedation and monitoring in our specialty. I am extremely pleased that Dr John Vargo agreed to be the guest editor for this issue. Dr Vargo, Chief of Gastroenterology and Hepatology at the Cleveland Clinic, has shown outstanding leadership in this field. His choice of topics and author-experts covers it all: preprocedural assessment, training and competency, legal issues, monitoring during endoscopy, special populations (including children, obesity, and sleep apnea), quality assurance, sedation in the Ambulatory Endoscopy Center, and computer-assisted and patient-controlled sedation. Finally, there is a topic looking into the future, which suggests the possibility of new drugs and methods that will bring improved safety and comfort at lower cost. This would be a dream come true. In the meantime, all gastrointestinal endoscopists should read this issue. It's a wake-up call.

Charles J. Lightdale, MD
Division of Digestive and Liver Diseases
Columbia University Medical Center
161 Fort Washington Avenue
New York, NY 10032, USA

E-mail address:
CJL18@columbia.edu

Preface

Sedation and Monitoring in Gastrointestinal Endoscopy

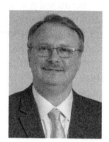

John J. Vargo, MD, MPH, AGAF, FACP, FACG, FASGE
Editor

There is a time for many words, and there is also a time for sleep.
　　　　　　　　　　　　　　　　　　—Homer, The Odyssey

This issue of *Gastrointestinal Endoscopy Clinics of North America* entitled, "Sedation and Monitoring in Gastrointestinal Endoscopy," deals with an element of our practice landscape that has changed dramatically over the past 10 years. In the last iteration of this topic in *Gastrointestinal Endoscopy Clinics of North America*, the majority of procedural sedation revolved around moderate sedation with a combination of a benzodiazepine and opioid that was delivered under the direction of the endoscopist. Exciting data on gastroenterologist-directed propofol sedation were coming to fruition with the promise of continued safety and satisfaction with vastly improved throughput parameters. How much things have changed in 10 years! Anesthetist-directed propofol sedation has literally and figuratively become the coin of the realm. In some areas of the country, gastroenterologists no longer practice procedural sedation and fellows graduate from their programs not being trained in this technique.

The following collection of articles provides a primer for the practitioner and trainee alike in addressing training and competency in sedation practice, the preprocedural assessment of the patient, the role of quality assurance in procedural sedation, how to achieve an important balance between safety and throughput in the endoscopy suite as well as an important discussion on risk management. The use of nonoperative remote anesthesia is discussed by a group of anesthesiologists who pioneered the role in the endoscopy suite many years ago and remain among the thought-leaders in their specialty. In addition, the role of procedural sedation in specialized populations such as children and in those with obesity and sleep apnea is addressed. We also look beyond pulse oximetry to extended monitoring technologies, such as capnography, and critically appraise their value. We review the role of

Gastrointest Endoscopy Clin N Am 26 (2016) xv–xvi
http://dx.doi.org/10.1016/j.giec.2016.04.002
1052-5157/16/$ – see front matter © 2016 Published by Elsevier Inc.

giendo.theclinics.com

computer-assisted sedation and revisit endoscopist-directed propofol sedation: will it ever regain its former foothold? Finally, we gaze into a crystal ball in an attempt to determine what procedural sedation for gastrointestinal endoscopy may look like in the future.

I am honored and humbled to have been given the privilege to edit this work. I would like to thank Dr Charlie Lightdale for the opportunity. His career of clinical care and research was a beacon to me as junior fellow and remains as such many years later. I would also like to thank the group of world-class authors who contributed to this issue. In closing, I would also like to remind our readers that complacency should never be in a clinician's lexicon. We all garner a sacred and unwavering responsibility to build upon our current practice of procedural sedation to make it more effective and safer in this evolving value-based practice environment.

John J. Vargo, MD, MPH, AGAF, FACP, FACG, FASGE
Cleveland Clinic
Digestive Disease Institute
Department of Gastroenterology and Hepatology
Desk A 30
9500 Euclid Avenue
Cleveland, OH 44195, USA

E-mail address:
vargoj@ccf.org

Preprocedural Assessment for Sedation in Gastrointestinal Endoscopy

John E. Tetzlaff, MD*, Walter G. Maurer, MD

KEYWORDS

- The "anesthesia approach to preparation" • The risk of complications • Sedation
- Hypoxemia • Aspiration • Cardiac disease • Pulmonary disease • Difficult airway

KEY POINTS

- Identification of the procedure planned.
- Define the goals for sedation for the planned procedure.
- Identify the comorbidity of the patients.
- Recognize the potential complications of sedation for endoscopic procedures.

INTRODUCTION

The role of the anesthesia service in sedation for gastrointestinal endoscopy (GIE) has been steadily increasing.[1,2] The goals of preprocedural assessment for GIE are determined by the specific details of the procedure, the issues related to the illness that requires the endoscopy, comorbidities, the goals for sedation, and the risk of complications from the sedation and the endoscopic procedure. Rather than consider these issues as separate entities, they should be considered as part of a continuum of preparation for GIE. This is told from the perspective of an anesthesiologist who regularly participates in the full range of sedation for the full spectrum of GIE.

THE ANESTHESIA APPROACH TO PREPARATION FOR A PROCEDURE

Because any anesthesia case can evolve in complexity, preparation focuses on the needs for the most complex. The starting point is a traditional history and physical (H&P) examination, with all additional interventions driven by the results.[3] The age and weight are the context, but do not dictate any specific testing. The present illness dictates further preparation, when there are interventions that delineate diminished

Cleveland Clinic Lerner College of Medicine of Case Western Reserve University, Department of General Anesthesia, Cleveland Clinic, 9500 Euclid Avenue, Cleveland, Ohio 44195, USA
* Corresponding author.
E-mail address: Tetzlaj@ccf.org

Gastrointest Endoscopy Clin N Am 26 (2016) 433–441
http://dx.doi.org/10.1016/j.giec.2016.02.001
1052-5157/16/$ – see front matter © 2016 Elsevier Inc. All rights reserved.

functional capacity, or by virtue of events, such as hemorrhage.[4] The comorbidities are identified in the context of how the disease influences functional reserves of major organs. The physical examination is targeted to the heart, lungs, central nervous system, and gastrointestinal (GI) tract with special attention to the airway. The penultimate element of preparation is the use of all of these elements to create a plan for the anesthetic intervention. For GIE, this would range from mild sedation to general anesthesia (GA). The plan requires realistic descriptions to the patient of the options for sedation and informed consent. For upper endoscopy, the invasiveness of upper endoscopy intubation requires either a cooperative or unconscious patient.[5] This is a key element of the plan as well as consent.

CONTRAST BETWEEN THE ENDOSCOPY SUITE AND THE OPERATING ROOM

In the operating room (OR), the surgeon is the primary care physician (PCP) for the patient, and directly or indirectly responsible for all elements of preparation, even those delegated to the anesthesia team. In contrast, many endoscopy suites are often open units, and the endoscopist is rarely the PCP. In the absence of protocols, many elements of preparation can be variable in this setting.[6] Even the basic H&P and preprocedural instructions may not occur without specific unit protocol. Preparation is limited to those measures that prepare the patient for endoscopy with little attention to preparation for an anesthetic intervention.[7] On the other hand, the conditions during endoscopy are different from surgery, where immobility, total anesthesia, and complete analgesic are assumed. During endoscopy with conscious sedation, some movement is the rule rather than the exception, and the discussion of approaches to sedation reflects this set point for both the patient and the endoscopist. Also, procedural amnesia is not always required during some GIEs. Inadequate preparation by the referring PCP that necessitates cancelling the case requires education of the PCP as to the needs for proper preparation to facilitate safe sedation for GIE.

GASTROINTESTINAL ENDOSCOPY PROCEDURES

Most GEI procedures (GIEPs) are esophagogastroduodenoscopy (EGD) or colonoscopy for diagnoses of benign conditions or cancer screening for healthy, ambulatory patients. The sedation needs are limited and the preparation is mainly determined by the needs of the endoscopy procedure. Physical preparation of the patient is the responsibility of the PCP or the physician ordering the endoscopy. Laboratory testing is unusual and nothing by mouth (NPO) intervals are short, accommodating the needs of the intestinal preparation, especially for colonoscopy. When a GIEP requires deep sedation or GA, this level of preparation may be inadequate. Participation or direction by the anesthesia team may improve efficiency of the endoscopy suite.[8,9]

With repeat procedures, the outcome of previous sedation can dictate the degree of preparation required. When the procedure is brief, the sedation minimal, and the patient satisfaction with the previous procedure high, minimal preparation is again reasonable. When the outcome is otherwise, deeper sedation may be necessary and more involved preparation and longer NPO intervals may be required. When the next procedure is more involved, such as endoscopic ultrasound (EUS) or endoscopic retrograde cholangiopancreatography (ERCP), the depth of sedation needed is deeper. The need for preparation is greater as is the need to inform the patient of the need for deeper sedation. If deep sedation or GA is required, the patient must be clearly informed of the correct NPO interval, especially if bowel preparation is required.

THE GASTROINTESTINAL ILLNESSES THAT REQUIRES ENDOSCOPY

An increasing number of patients require these routine GIEs for various chronic GI diseases, such as Crohn disease, Barrett esophagus, or ulcerative colitis, and may require sedation administered by an anesthesia team for patient comfort or safety. These patients may need to be prepared in a manner analogous to the process used before ambulatory surgery. A subset of these patients will require formal GA for which preparation is directed by the need for GA.[10]

When GI bleeding is involved,[11] preparation is directed toward anemia. With chronic anemia, the minimum hemoglobin level allowable for deep sedation or GA is considered to be approximately 8 g/dL. In the setting of acute GI bleeding with deep endoscopy (double-balloon, single-balloon, or spiral endoscopy), deep sedation or GA may be required.[12] Acute hemorrhage in the face of myocardial or cerebral ischemia may require higher hemoglobin levels for sedation. The availability of blood is best determined by a type and screen that could identify any problems, such as the presence of antibodies. This could adversely affect quick availability of blood products.

ALTERED GASTROINTESTINAL MOTILITY

When GI mobility is decreased, preparation for sedation is dictated by the risk of aspiration. With gastroparesis or achalasia, dietary restrictions may need to be extended and NPO intervals for liquids 8 hours or greater. With gastric outlet obstruction, the potential full stomach may require GA with endotracheal intubation. This is also true with anticipated tight esophageal stricture, where residual liquid or solid may be encountered. Preparation may extend to the approach to upper endoscopy, with a small endoscope and topical anesthesia allowing entry to the esophagus and stomach. If empty, the procedure proceeds. If high liquid gastric or esophageal residual is encountered, one of the choices is to empty the liquid with endoscopic suction and proceed. If excessive liquid or solid residual is encountered, the endoscope is withdrawn and either intubation of the trachea to protect from aspiration or terminate the procedure and reschedule after a longer liquid diet regimen are the options. Although clear liquids have the fastest transit time, and all colonoscopy preparation solutions are clear liquids, their large volumes can affect the residual left in the stomach if they are consumed right before the procedure and increase the risk of regurgitation, which could cause aspiration.

INFECTION

When the indication for the endoscopy is infection (abscess, cholangitis), the goal of preparation for sedation is to determine if the patient is hemodynamically stable. Signs of sepsis include fever, hypotension, and tachycardia. Laboratory investigation should focus on identification of leukocytosis and metabolic acidosis. Optimization requires antibiotic administration and correction of intravascular volume deficits, as hypovolemia can cause hemodynamic instability during sedation.

BILIARY AND PANCREATIC DISEASES

Most of the endoscopy procedures involving the biliary tract require advanced endoscopic techniques, such as ERCP or EUS[13] with deep sedation, which dictates preparation for anesthesia delivered service. Procedures that involve common duct obstructions can be associated with cholangitis with liberation of purulent material into the proximal upper GI tract and may require general endotracheal anesthesia (GETA). Copious stones in the ductal system may require high-volume irrigation, which creates the potential for regurgitation of liquid that exceeds the performance of endo-scopic suction with the potential of pulmonary aspiration, also requiring GETA. Drainage of large pancreatic cysts also may overwhelm endoscopic suction, with the potential for infected pulmonary aspiration, another indication of GETA. EUS-guided biopsy of the pancreas may be more successful with anesthesia-directed deep sedation.[14]

COMORBIDITY

The impact of comorbidity is determined by the disease, the severity of the disease, and the compliance of the individual with treatment. The combination of these factors measures the functional capacity of the patient, which in turn predicts the response of the patient to depth of sedation. In general, the better the functional capacity, the less likely the complications of deep sedation.

Cardiovascular Diseases

Poorly controlled hypertension can present issues for GIE because of the varying levels if stimulus during the procedures. The endoscopic intubation can be stimulating, as can various maneuvers during the procedure.[15] This can occur in patients who are very dependent on their antihypertensive, and who may receive varying instructions. Without proper instructions, many hypertensive patients will avoid taking their hyper-tensive medications. The result can be stimulus from endoscopy, no medication, and light sedation, creating very high blood pressures. The opposite extreme is equally true with sedation causing vasodilation synergistic to antihypertensive medications taken on the morning of surgery and precipitous drops in blood pressure, with a loss of consciousness. There is no universal agreement for the definition of controlled versus uncontrolled hypertension, but starting systolic pressure greater than 180 mm Hg should raise concern. For structural heart disease, the entities most likely to occur are coronary artery disease, valvular heart disease (VHD), cardiomyopathy (CM), or congestive heart failure (CHF). Without the input of the anesthesia team, the assump-tion about GIE is that there is minimal interaction with cardiac disease, which could not be further from the truth.[15] NPO status, bowel preparation, and sympathetic stimula-tion can present during sedation as tachycardia, arrhythmia and/or hypotension. Compliance with cardiac medications is important, as in correct instructions about the myriad of anticoagulant medication prescribed for various aspects of cardiovascu-lar disease.[11] For VHD, stenotic valves are more difficult to manage than the regurgi-tant values and identifying critical aortic or mitral stenosis is an important element of preparation for sedation.[15] When faced with a patient who has a critically stenotic valvular lesion with an urgent indication for GIE, it is important to plan to maintain homeostasis, avoiding wide swings in blood pressure, heart rate, and oxygen satura-tion. The decision between deep sedation and GETA in a patient with tight aortic stenosis is modified by the sympathetic stimulation induced by endotracheal intuba-tion, which can be avoided when sedation with spontaneous ventilation is chosen. Obstructive CM can behave like a stenotic heart valve lesion and amyl nitrate during echocardiography can reveal very high pressure gradients that also can be induced during sedation when hypovolemic.

The basic history and physical may reveal symptoms indicative of diminished cardiac reserves, such as chest pain, shortness of breath (SOB), or diminished activity tolerance. Twelve-lead electrocardiogram is indicated with history of structural heart disease. Further investigations can reveal an indication for transthoracic echocardiog-raphy for VHD, such as syncope, murmur associated with dizziness, or SOB with minimal exertion. If myocardial ischemia is suspected, a functional study such as a cardiac stress test may be indicated. If the patient arrives for GIE with any of these issues without investigation, proceeding will carry increased risk or will need to be postponed until further cardiac evaluation is completed. When bleeding is the indication for the GIE, stress testing may be deferred because the outcome of a positive test would be angiography, which in turn would be contraindicated because any intervention would require anticoagulation.

Pulmonary Disease

Diminished pulmonary reserves directly interact with sedation for upper endoscopy because of the interference with ventilation, which in turn can further compromise oxygenation. Sedatives for GIE sedation have in common some degree of respiratory depression and events like coughing, hiccups, pooled secretion and or laryngospasm can acutely accentuate any existing respiratory depression. In addition, endoscopic techniques impose temporary burdens on the respiratory system from insufflation, particularly when carbon dioxide is used.[16–20]

The assessment of pulmonary reserves is focused around the history and physical. For the history element, activity tolerance is the focus with SOB, limited activity tolerance, and the need for supplemental oxygen at rest being key. Recognition of obstructive sleep apnea (OSA) is important, as the presence of OSA predicts some issues with tolerance of sedation.[21] If the patient can walk reasonable distances, or tolerate moderate exertion, sedation for upper endoscopy can be induced with careful control of the sedative levels and avoidance of respiratory depression. For this reason, opioids are added to the sedative mixture with caution. If activity is limited to a few steps or supplemental oxygen is required at rest, mild to moderate sedation can be dangerous and a full anesthesia intervention, including endotracheal intubation may be needed. An alternative is excellent topical anesthesia and light sedation before upper endoscopy if a simple and brief procedure is planned. Rarely formal evaluation by a pulmonologist with formal pulmonary function testing can be indicated for optimization of a patient with limited pulmonary reserves who needs an elective advanced endoscopy procedure.

Neurologic Diseases

The interface between preparation for GIE and neurologic disease focuses around issues of diminished GI motility with decreased gastric and proximal intestinal emptying and risk of aspiration. Dietary habits, swallowing impairment, decreased gag reflex, early satiety, and nausea and/or vomiting are important indications that increased gastric residual of liquid or solid food present a risk of pulmonary aspiration. This in turn dictates that the procedure must be performed either with intact airway reflects or an airway secured by an endotracheal tube.

Renal Disease

Chronic renal disease will impact sedation for GIE when the patient is oliguric or dialysis-dependent related to volume status and/or electrolyte disturbance. The need for bowel preparation can accentuate these issues by virtue of further volume loss and electrolyte disturbance. When possible, a dialysis patient should be scheduled for GIE on the days between dialysis sessions. If scheduled immediately before dialysis, there can be volume overload and solute accumulation (hyperkalemia). If scheduled immediately after dialysis, postdialysis shock related to too much or too little fluid and/or acute electrolyte disturbances is an issue. The combination of structural cardiac disease with end-stage renal disease can present a particularly difficult patient to sedate. Hypoventilation or insufflation with CO_2 can create acidosis and subsequently, further increase hyperkalemia, if present.

Airway Examination

An essential element of preparation for sedation for GIEP is detection of potential issues that predict difficult airway management or hypoxemia.[22] Obese patients require a focused airway examination to detect signs that predict difficult airway management.[23] OSA is being increasingly recognized as a risk for hypoxemia and diminished pulmonary reserves. Identifying symptoms, such as snoring, periodic breathing, or daytime sleepiness, can identify a subset of patients for sedation who may be at risk for complications. Questionnaires designed to identify OSA, such as Stop-Bang can be useful. A full face, thick neck, or beard may represent a patient with difficult mask ventilation, which in turn reflects on the degree of difficulty with airway rescue during sedation.

The formal airway examination includes the Mallampati classification, lip-bite test, range of motion of the neck, thyromental distance, mouth opening, and neck circumferences. Not every patient with indicators of difficult intubation needs to be intubated for GIE, but part of preparation for these patients involves consideration of the anesthesia team involvement in their sedation and recovery, in the event that airway compromise occurs. At minimum, there must be skilled personnel immediately available to institute airway interventions, and in this subset of patients, the availability of airway management skill is an element of preparation.[24,25] Upper endoscopy with sedation in a patient with OSA who seems to have good respirations during the procedure may become problematic in the postanesthesia care unit, especially with residual sedation, because during the procedure, the OSA is usually alleviated by the airway being improved with the endoscope.

THE GOALS OF SEDATION

Part of the preparation for sedation is the informed consent, matching the depth of sedation with the expectations of the patient. This is in contrast with OR cases, when the default is unconsciousness, complete anesthesia, and analgesia. The range of patient expectations for sedation during GIE is wide. Some patients undergoing brief diagnostic endoscopy will prefer to remain alert with topical anesthesia for comfort. The opposite extreme is the patient who insists on GA, regardless of the endoscopic procedure. The fallacy in preparation for sedation is the assumption that the degree of preparation is determined by the depth of sedation. The mistake is to assume that less sedation requires less preparation. This becomes an error when the depth of sedation increases and minor consequences interact with elements not considered during preparation. This is particularly true with cardiac and or pulmonary comorbidity during unanticipated deep sedation, where hemodynamic instability and or hypoxemia/hypercarbia can require management and worst case, create morbidity.

At times, the goals for sedation can be dictated by previous experiences with endoscopy procedures. Either pain with upper or lower endoscopy or gagging/retching with upper endoscopy can create intense fear of being conscious during subsequent endoscopy. Part of preparing these patients for GIE may be planning for deeper sedation than is indicated by the procedure. This is also true when a prior procedure could not be completed because stimulation made it necessary to abort the procedure. Moderate or deep sedation may allow completion of various endoscopy maneuvers, such as intubation of the cecum.[26] It may also be indicated when a lesion is encountered that requires a more extensive procedure. All of these scenarios demand realistic informed consent such that sedation delivered accomplishes the goals and meets the patient's expectations.

COMPLICATIONS OF SEDATION FOR GASTROINTESTINAL ENDOSCOPY

The goals for sedation also can be dictated by the GI pathology. A brief EGD has different sedation goals when gastroparesis, achalasia, or gastric outlet obstruction is known. Preparation for a full general endotracheal anesthetic is wise, even if not initially planned. Even mild depression of respiration with light sedation may induce hypoxemia when severe decrease in respiratory reserve is present. The ability to intubate, control respiration, and maintain controlled ventilation after the procedure are reasonable elements of preparation. Use of opioids can be a reasonable choice for routine or advanced GIE, but must be selected with caution or avoided in the patient with OSA. Unrecognized OSA should be considered. The mild stimulation of upper or lower GIE for surveillance or to rule out occult GI bleeding must be handled when it is a preoperative procedure before aortic valve replacement in a patient with critical aortic stenosis. Even bowel preparation can be a traumatic intervention in a patient with symptomatic obstruction cardiomyopathy who will poorly tolerate any degree of hypovolemia, which induces cardiac outflow obstruction. This is also true for patients with poorly compensated CHF. Even mild anemia can require careful transfusion of red cells before endoscopy treatment of GI hemorrhage in a patient with inducible myocardial ischemia. Any GIE can require surgical or interventional radiology procedures when complications such as perforation or uncontrolled bleeding occur and make preprocedural preparation an element of patient safety.

SUMMARY

The goals for preprocedural preparation for sedation during GIE are determined by the specific procedure planned, the GI pathology, other comorbidity, the goals of the sedation, and some anticipated complications. Comorbidity in cardiac, pulmonary, neurologic, and renal disease can create issues for sedation that require preparation. GI disease, such as bleeding, decreased gastric or esophageal emptying, stricture, or the need to irrigate stones or drain a pancreatic pseudocyst, may dictate deep sedation or GETA, which requires informed consent for the sedation technique and other preparation as patient health status dictates. Even routine surveillance GIE can require extensive preparation when they are screening procedures for cardiac transplantation or other open heart surgery. Likewise, the brief GIE can be challenging in patients with severely decreased pulmonary reserves. Even small doses of opioids as an element of procedural sedation can have exaggerated impact with respiratory depression in patients with severe OSA and OSA should be considered as a possible etiology in patients difficult to sedate.

REFERENCES

1. Liu H, Waxman DA, Main R, et al. Utilization of anesthesia services during outpatient endoscopies and colonoscopies and associated spending in 2003-2009. JAMA 2012;307:1178–84.
2. Alharbi O, Rabeneck L, Paszat LF, et al. A population-based analysis of outpatient colonoscopy in adults assisted by an anesthesiologist. Anesthesiology 2009;111:734–40.

3. Hausman LM, Reich DL. Providing safe sedation/analgesia: anesthesiologist's perspective. Gastrointest Endosc Clin N Am 2008;18:707–16.
4. deVilliers WJ. Anesthesiology and gastroenterology. Anesthesiol Clin 2009;27: 57–70.
5. Barriga J, Sachdev MS, Royall L, et al. Sedation for upper endoscopy: comparison of midazolam versus fentanyl plus midazolam. South Med J 2008;101:362–6.
6. Goulson DT, Fragneto RY. Anesthesia for gastrointestinal endoscopic procedures. Anesthesiol Clin 2009;27:71–85.
7. Cohen LB, DeLegge MH, Aisenberg J, et al. AGA institute review of endoscopic sedation. Gastroenterology 2007;133:675–701.
8. Aisenberg J, Cohen LB. Sedation in endoscopic practice. Gastrointest Endosc Clin N Am 2006;16:695–708.
9. Shah B, Cohen LB. The changing faces of endoscopic sedation. Expert Rev Gastroenterol Hepatol 2010;4:417–22.
10. Trummel J. Sedation for gastrointestinal endoscopy: the changing landscape. Curr Opin Anaesthesiol 2007;20:359–64.
11. Wassef W, Rukkan R. Interventional endoscopy. Curr Opin Gastroenterol 2005;21: 644–52.
12. Shah N, Vargo JJ. Basic requirements of gastroenterologists to treat gastrointestinal bleeding: competency and sedation issues. Gastrointest Endosc Clin N Am 2011;21:731–7.
13. Albashir S, Stevens T. Endoscopic ultrasonography to evaluate pancreatitis. Cleve Clin J Med 2012;79:202–6.
14. Ootaki C, Stevens ST, Vargo J, et al. Does general anesthesia increase the diagnostic yield of endoscopic ultrasound-guided fine needle aspiration of pancreatic masses. Anesthesiology 2012;117:1044–50.
15. Ross C, Fishman WH, Peterson SJ, et al. Cardiovascular considerations in patients undergoing gastrointestinal endoscopy. Cardiol Rev 2008;16:76–81.
16. Suzuki T, Minami H, Komatsu T, et al. Prolonged carbon dioxide insufflation under general anesthesia for endoscopic submucosal dissection. Endoscopy 2010;42: 1021–9.
17. Takano A, Kobayaski M, Tacheuchi M, et al. Capnographic monitoring during endoscopic submucosal dissection with patients under deep sedation: a prospective crossover trial of air and carbon dioxide insufflations. Digestion 2011; 84:193–8.
18. Bretthauer M, Selp B, Ausen S, et al. Carbon dioxide insufflation for more comfortable endoscopic retrograde cholangiopancreatography: a randomized double blind trial. Endoscopy 2007;39:68–74.
19. Dellon ES, Hawk JS, Grimm IS, et al. The use of carbon dioxide for insufflation during GI endoscopy: a systematic review. Gastrointest Endosc 2009;69:843–9.
20. Janssens F, Deviere J, Eisendrath P, et al. Carbon dioxide for gut distension during digestive endoscopy: technique and practice survey. World J Gastroenterol 2009;15:1475–9.
21. Waugh JB, Epps CA, Khodneva YA. Capnography enhances surveillance of respiratory events during procedural sedation: a meta-analysis. J Clin Anesth 2011; 23:189–96.
22. Vargo J. Sedation in the bariatric patient. Gastrointest Endosc Clin N Am 2011;21: 257–63.
23. Schreiner MA, Fennerty MB. Endoscopy in the obese patient. Gastroenterol Clin North Am 2010;39:87–97.

24. Cote GA, Houis RM, Ansstas MA, et al. Incidence of sedation-related complications with propofol use during advanced endoscopic procedures. Clin Gastroenterol Hepatol 2010;8:137–42.
25. American Society of Anesthesiologists Task Force on Sedation and Analgesia by Non-Anesthesiologists. Practice guidelines for sedation and analgesia by non-anesthesiologists. Anesthesiology 2002;96:1004–17.
26. Chelazzi C, Gonsales G, Boninsegni P, et al. Propofol sedation in a colorectal cancer screening outpatient cohort. Minerva Anestesiol 2009;75:677–83.

Training and Competency in Sedation Practice in Gastrointestinal Endoscopy

Ben Da, MD, James Buxbaum, MD*

KEYWORDS

- Conscious sedation • Deep sedation • Endoscopy • Gastrointestinal • Curriculum
- Education • Medical • Graduate

KEY POINTS

- Instruction in endoscopic sedation includes theoretical and practice-based components.
- Critical skills needed to safely perform sedation include preprocedural assessment, informed consent, sedation administration, intraprocedure and postprocedure monitoring, adverse event management, and safe discharge.
- The use of propofol by nonanesthesia providers mandates a more intense training curriculum given the narrow therapeutic range and resulting increased risk of deep or general anesthesia induction.
- Simulation allows trainees to gain hands-on experience managing sedation and related adverse events in a controlled environment.
- Methods to assess endoscopic sedation competency differ among institutions, but requires testing of knowledge and technical skills.

NEED FOR SEDATION TRAINING

The purpose of endoscopic sedation is to relieve the patient's discomfort and anxiety while simultaneously reducing disruptive movements so that an adequate endoscopic examination may be performed. Patient safety needs to be ensured while procedural efficacy is maintained. The delivery of sedation requires multifaceted expertise and the endoscopist needs to be adept at each step of the sedation process ranging from preprocedural planning to patient discharge.[1,2]

The increasing use of propofol to support endoscopy has intensified awareness of these challenges.[3–13] Although large studies have demonstrated consistently low

Disclosures: The authors have no relevant conflict of interest to disclose.
Division of Gastroenterology and Liver Diseases, Keck School of Medicine, University of Southern California, Los Angeles, CA, USA
* Corresponding author. Keck School of Medicine, University of Southern California, D & T Building Room B4H100, 1983 Marengo Street, Los Angeles, CA 90033-1370.
E-mail address: jbuxbaum@usc.edu

morbidity, the classification of this agent as a general anesthetic has led to questions about endoscopists' lack of proper training in sedation and potential ramifications for patient safety.[14,15] Furthermore, a significant portion of the American malpractice claims against gastroenterologists originates from sedation-related complications.[16,17]

Thus, a key challenge currently encountered in fellowship programs and clinical institutions is to ensure that endoscopists are trained properly in the practice of sedation to the level of competency. Traditionally, training in sedation for endoscopy has been done via the informal apprentice and mentor model within the endoscopy suite.[18–20] Although training under the direct guidance of an anesthesiologist has not been required, the consensus of the gastroenterology community is that the training process needs to be done with a more thorough and programmatic approach.[17,20–23] This process includes the need for formal education, simulator-based experiences, immediately supervised hands-on practice, and finally testing for competence.[1] In this review, we aim to cover the current guidelines and approaches to training gastroenterologists in the practice of sedation and the tools available for assessing competency.

CURRENT GUIDELINES

The most widely recognized American curriculum and competency guidelines for sedation training of Gastroenterology professionals are included in the Multisociety Sedation Curriculum for Gastrointestinal Endoscopy (MSCGE; 2012) derived from the combined efforts of the American Society for Gastrointestinal Endoscopy, American Gastroenterological Association, American College of Gastroenterology, the American Association for the Study of Liver Disease, and the Society for Gastroenterology Nurses and Associates.[1,2,17] The American Society of Anesthesiologists (ASA) sedation guidelines for nonanesthesiologists (2002) remains highly influential.[2] The most recent European curriculum comes from a consortium of the European Society of Gastrointestinal Endoscopy, European Society of Gastroenterology, and the European Society of and Gastroenterology and Endoscopy Nurses and Associates in 2013.[23] This curriculum was updated in 2015 with a special focus on nonanesthesiologist administered propofol training.[24] Other published guidelines include the Spanish Society of Digestive Endoscopy (2014), Japanese Gastroenterological Endoscopy (2015), Australian Tripartite Endoscopy Sedation Committee (2010), and the German (S3; 2008) guidelines.[2,22,25–28] The impact of the implementation of the S3 guidelines has been the subject of prospective investigation.[29]

Although the guidelines differ in specific content, they emphasize that the training process needs to include both theoretical and practical skills training.[1,23] The former involves a blend of didactics and self-teaching and the latter entails simulation scenarios as well as direct observation of clinical performance by an instructor. The 2 main curricula defer in that the MSCGE takes a more self-directed, individualized approach to learning, whereas the European curriculum serves as more of an instruction guide to teachers and organizations seeking to organize sedation courses. The MSCGE aims to provide a foundation of knowledge and then create pathways to allow the individual to fill in gaps in their current understanding of endoscopic sedation.[1,23] The course structure of the European curriculum consists of a 3-day introductory course that combines theory and practice followed by at least a 2-week course of clinical training with a mentor.[23] Both courses recommend detailed training in preprocedure assessment and preparation, appropriate pharmacologic and monitoring strategies during the procedure, management of adverse events, and postprocedure monitoring.[1,23]

TRAINING IN PREPROCEDURE MANAGEMENT

Training in sedation preparation involves learning how to perform an adequate risk assessment and determining when to enlist the assistance of an anesthesia professional. This should be done congruently with other pre-endoscopic evaluations, such as the need for antibiotic prophylaxis and bleeding tendency.[30] In the United States, fellowship trainees are required to complete institution-specific written or computerized case-based models on sedation risk assessment.[31] However, almost the entirety of their training occurs through "on-the-job" training during faculty-supervised endoscopy.[18–20]

Risk Assessment

Training to perform an accurate risk assessment begins with learning how to conduct a careful history and focused physical examination. The trainee needs to assess for a previous adverse reaction to sedatives, symptoms of obstructive sleep apnea, and a history of alcohol overuse or drug abuse.[2,17] These risk factors are associated with sedation complications.[32–35] The physical examination should focus on vital signs, mental status, and the presence of pathologic anatomic features associated with a greater risk of airway obstruction such as craniofacial malformation, tumors, or restricted mouth opening. The trainee needs to be able to apply the Mallampati scoring system to predict ease of intubation.[36] Cardiopulmonary findings such as wheezing or crackles suggest the presence of underlying asthma or fluid overload. The anticipated complexity of the planned procedure may also contribute to this risk profile and preprocedure management.[37] For example, some facilities mandate that all patients undergoing high complexity procedures such as endoscopic retrograde cholangiopancreatography be sedated by the anesthesia service.[38]

The trainee needs to be able to use the ASA physical status classification.[36,39] Although endoscopist-directed sedation is usually safe for patients with an ASA class of II or lower, increasing ASA scores positively correlates with a higher rate of sedation complications and requirement for emergency reversal strategies.[40–45] Various guidelines differ regarding which ASA class is considered high risk for sedation. American guidelines consider physical class IV or higher to have severe systemic disease and suggest an anesthesiologist to manage sedation.[1,17,39] The S3 endoscopic sedation guidelines from Germany emphasize patients of class of III or higher are at higher risk for sedation. After the completion of a 3-day training program based on the S3 guidelines, the use of the ASA classification to classify patient risk increased by more than 20% across 224 German institutions.[46]

Special Circumstances

The practice of endoscopic sedation in the pregnant and elderly population warrants discussion during the training process.[1] Endoscopy and the use of sedation should not be used in pregnancy unless absolutely necessary because the fetus may be exposed to hypoxemia and hypotension during the use of endoscopic sedation, which can potentially lead to fetal injury.[1] Certain medications including benzodiazepines are contraindicated in pregnancy. When performing endoscopic sedation on an elderly patient, increased attention needs to be paid to the presence of age-related diseases (eg, cardiac dysfunction), enhanced sensitivity to sedatives, increased risk of aspiration, and prolonged recovery time.[47] During training, endoscopists should practice decreasing the risk associated with sedation by using only a portion of the recommended initial dose, minimizing the total dose given, and slowly titrating sedatives during the procedure.[48,49] A more detailed discussion of the preprocedure assessment of high-risk patients is included in a dedicated section of this edition of *Gastrointestinal Endoscopy Clinics of North America*. Ultimately, the decision of whether a gastroenterologist should perform the sedation or defer to an anesthesiologist comes from taking all risk factors into consideration.

Obtaining Informed Consent and Documentation

Despite being a critical part of the preprocedure assessment with the ability to mitigate malpractice risk, a significant proportion of gastroenterology fellowship programs do not offer structured training in informed consent.[19,50] Obtaining proper informed consent for endoscopic sedation is an underrecognized part of the preprocedural assessment. Sedation represents a significant portion of the complications related to performing endoscopy and in many medicolegal cases patients attested that they were inadequately aware of nonprocedural risks.[51,52] The trainee must be able to determine that the patient is competent enough to give consent.[53] After establishing competency, the trainee must then accurately explain what endoscopic sedation entails to inform the patient to make an autonomous decision. This includes information regarding the benefits, risks, and alternatives of sedation including the options for anesthesiologist-delivered sedation or unsedated endoscopy.[24,54] Careful documentation of informed consent is now the standard. The ability to properly perform documentation of other vital information (eg, vital signs, home medications) and time out before the procedure is also expected of the trainee before the start of independent practice.[1,17,23]

TRAINING IN SEDATION ADMINISTRATION
Level of Sedation

After the preprocedure assessment training is done, the trainee then needs to learn the differences between the different levels of sedation and how to determine which level is ideal for different procedures and situations. Minimal and moderate sedation still leaves the patient able to respond purposefully to actions and commands while cardiovascular and ventilation functions are still preserved. Deep and general sedation represents a continuum in which patients may require assistance with maintaining airway or cardiovascular function (**Table 1**).[45,55] General anesthesia is strictly the domain of anesthesia specialists who can perform complex maneuvers to maintain adequate respiration and cardiovascular function.[26] In most situations, the endoscopist's goal is to achieve moderate sedation successfully. However, a trainee should recognize that the boundary between moderate and deep sedation is often vague and thus should be prepared to manage patients that transiently become deeply sedated.[1] Trainees must be cognizant that all sedative agents they use can result in general anesthesia.[17]

To monitor and quantify a patient's level of sedation, trainees should be aware of the available validated scoring systems. The most frequently used scale is the Observer's Assessment of Alertness/Sedation (OAA/S) (**Table 2**). Other scoring systems include the Sedation-Agitation Scale (SAS), Ramsay Sedation Scale, and the Modified Richmond Agitation-Sedation Score.[56–59] Upper endoscopies and colonoscopies can usually be managed by moderate sedation, whereas longer and more complex procedures like endoscopic retrograde cholangiopancreatography or endoscopic ultrasound examinations may require deep sedation or general anesthesia.[24,26,40,60,61] The use of deep sedation by endoscopists is controversial because there is concern that endoscopists lack the training to recognize and rescue a patient who loses their protective reflexes.[15]

Table 1
Continuum of sedation

	Minimal Sedation (Anxiolysis)	Moderate Sedation (Conscious Sedation)	Deep Sedation	General Anesthesia
Responsiveness	Normal response to verbal stimulation	Purposeful response to verbal or tactile stimulation	Purposeful response after repeated or painful stimulation	Unarousable, even with painful stimulus
Airway	Unaffected	No intervention required	Intervention may be required	Intervention often required
Spontaneous ventilation	Unaffected	Adequate	May be inadequate	Frequently inadequate
Cardiovascular function	Unaffected	Usually maintained	Usually maintained	May be impaired

Data from American Society of Anesthesiologists Task Force on Sedation and Analgesia by Non-Anesthesiologists. Practice guidelines for sedation and analgesia by non-anesthesiologists. Anesthesiology 2002;96:1004–17.

Table 2
Modified Observer's Assessment of Alertness/Sedation scale

Responsiveness	Numerical Score
Responds readily to name spoken in normal tone	5
Lethargic response to name spoken in normal tone	4
Responds only after name is called loudly and/or repeatedly	3
Responds only after mild prodding or shaking	2
Responds only after painful trapezius squeeze	1
No response after painful trapezius squeeze	0

Pharmacology and Medication Administration

Trainees need to recognize the appropriate agents, dosing, and timing of sedation medications to administer during endoscopy. The MSCGE advocates for both a cognitive training in medication management involving lectures and independent study as well as a procedure training portion that is bilevel.[1] The first component of hands-on procedure training involves the observation of a faculty member administering sedation and the use of a sedation simulator. Subsequently, the trainee should administer sedation under direct faculty supervision. Ideally, hands-on training is followed by case review sessions to discuss cases and adverse events.

Factors that should be considered when choosing sedation medications not only include type and expected duration of the procedure, but also patient-specific considerations including drug–drug interactions, side effects, and intolerance (**Table 3**).[2,23] Institutional regulations as well as state and national statutes may also impact the

Table 3
Pharmacologic profile of commonly used sedation agents

Drug	Onset of Action (min)	Peak Effect (min)	Duration of Effect (min)	Side Effects	Antagonism
Midazolam	1–2	3–4	15–80	Respiratory depression Disinhibition reactions Cardiac dysrhythmia	Flumazenil
Diazepam	2–3	3–5	360	Respiratory depression Disinhibition reactions	Flumazenil
Propofol	<1	1–2	4–8	Hypoxemia Apnea Hypotension Bradycardia Upper airway obstruction Injection site pain Propofol infusion syndrome	None
Meperidine	3–6	5–7	60–180	Synergistic respiratory depression Cardiovascular instability Nausea and vomiting Neurotoxicity with renal failure	Naloxone
Fentanyl	1–2	3–5	30–60	Synergistic respiratory depression Chest wall rigidity Skeletal muscle hypertonicity	Naloxone

Data from Refs.[1,17,66,97,122]

availability of certain agents. The induction and maintenance of sedation is a dynamic process that requires the trainee to continuously evaluate the depth of sedation, assess how the patient is tolerating the procedure, and recognize when the assistance of an anesthesia professional may be required emergently. More intensive training in sedation techniques, obtained through intensive care and anesthesia rotations, correlates with a decreased reliance of on fixed medication administration protocols (ie, scheduled doses every 3–5 minutes) and improved moderate sedation morbidity.[62]

Endoscopists have been traditionally the most comfortable with the use of the benzodiazepines and opiates combination as both medications have readily available reversal agents.[63] Benzodiazepines induce sedative, amnestic, and anxiolytic effects by activating the gamma-amino butyric acid receptor.[28] Midazolam is the benzodiazepine most often used in practice owing to its potency, relatively short half-life (2–6 hours), and amnesic properties. However, this medication still carries a significant rate of respiratory depression.[64–68] Opiates exert strong analgesic effects via the μ−opioid receptor. Fentanyl is favored owing to its combination of high potency, rapid onset, and short half-life (2–7 hours), which favors quicker recovery.[28] Opiates induce respiratory depression, particularly when given in combination with benzodiazepines.

Additional medications used in combination with benzodiazepines and opiates include antihistamines such as diphenhydramine and dopamine receptor antagonists including promethazine. However, the addition of these medications may increase the risk of hypoventilation and prolong recovery.[69,70] Ketamine and droperidol have also been used as adjuncts but the ketamine may result in an unpleasant psychological reaction and the droperidol has a US Food and Drug Administration black box warning for prolongation of QT intervals.[71,72]

Propofol

Propofol's favorable pharmacodynamic and pharmacokinetic profile (half-life of 2–4 minutes, onset of action <1 minute) has led to its widespread using in endoscopic sedation.[17,73] Propofol as a monotherapy in basic and advanced endoscopy has been shown to induce moderate sedation more rapidly than the midazolam and fentanyl or meperidine combinations, while improving recovery time and patient satisfaction in several randomized trials.[9,68,74–76] However, although the overall risk of adverse sedation events in large endoscopic series has been shown to be low, propofol has a much narrower window between moderate sedation and general anesthesia then benzodiazepines and narcotics.[10,27,28,77,78] Additionally, there is no reversal agent that can be administered if oversedation or loss of protective airway reflexes occurs. Thus, the US Food and Drug Administration has labeled propofol as a general anesthetic. A petition to change the warning labeling on propofol by the American College of Gastroenterology in 2010 was denied. Recently, the 21 European Anesthesiology Societies issued a consensus statement that nonanesthesiologists should not administer propofol.[14] However, the use of dedicated anesthesia providers to provide sedation for endoscopic procedures is costly and may not be financially feasible.[79,80]

In this controversial setting, guidelines recommend that nonanesthesiologists who administers propofol undergo more structured training and certification than those who administer strictly moderate sedation.[15] Typically this consists of institution-specific training courses and direct hands-on training with an anesthesiologist or another provider with more than 300 cases of propofol sedation experience.[23] For example, at Denmark's Gentofte University Hospital, a 6-week course was developed for nurse-administered propofol sedation (NAPS) sedation, which included rigorous training in practical airway management, observation, simulation training in adverse event management, and direct supervision.[61] The performance of the NAPS teams during the first 1764 cases after training was assessed by dividing them into 4 temporal quartiles of 441 patients. They requested assistance 8 times during the first quartile but only twice over the next 3 quartiles. Hypotension occurred in 73.2% of cases in the first quartile but in less than 15% in the third and fourth quartiles. Hypoxemia occurred in 4.4% and hypotension in 26%; however, all episodes responded to therapy and none of the procedures were cancelled. The authors concluded that with proper training NAPS is safe for endoscopic procedures. However, given that most challenges occurred during the first quartile, they did qualify that further training in administering propofol would have been helpful and at minimum an anesthesia provider should be available during the first 3 months of implementation (which was the case at their center). In Switzerland, there are also very active NAPS programs and the method of sedation for the majority of procedures is propofol administered by a nonanesthesiologist provider.[81]

Intraprocedural Monitoring

In addition to patient comfort, sedation strategy is driven by changes in vital parameters. Trainees must be able to interpret and respond to continuous pulse oximetry values.[20,63] The importance of continuous low-flow supplemental oxygen via the nasal or oral route (which prevents hypoxemia) on pulse oximetry values needs to be understood by trainees.[82–85] The frequency of monitoring additional vital signs, most importantly blood pressure, must be correlated to the patient's level of sedation.[1] After the introduction of a national endoscopic sedation curriculum and guideline in Germany, the use of routine supplemental oxygen increased from 34% to 64% and the use of automated blood pressure systems increased by 11%.[86] Although the monitoring of pulse oximetry and automated noninvasive blood pressure measurements are sufficient for most patients, an electrocardiogram should be used in patients with a history of cardiac or pulmonary disease.[17,23] After training, the trainee must be competent in identifying hypoxemia, hypotension, cardiac arrhythmias, and apnea.[1,2,23] Implementation of the S3 sedation training curriculum and guidelines resulted in a 2-fold increase in the use of periprocedural electrocardiography.[86]

Pulse oximetry is useful for detecting hypoxemia but has the limitation of being unable to measure hypercarbia, a sign of early hypoventilation.[87] Capnography, which uses infrared spectrography to provide a real-time graphic assessment of CO_2, is used routinely for this assessment. Vargo and colleagues[88] showed that pulse oximetry did not detect 50% of the apnea or disordered respiration episodes that capnography was able identify. However, capnography has only been shown to be of benefit in preventing hypoxemia in the pediatric population undergoing moderate sedation and in lengthier procedures like endoscopic retrograde cholangiopancreatography and endoscopic ultrasound examinations.[87,89] A University of Arizona practice project improved the understanding of capnography among nurses through interventions including staff education and nursing protocols.[90] Trainees should also be aware of the emergence of new technologies including the use of an electroencephalogram and the bispectral index for degree of sedation monitoring.[31] The bispectral index is a quantitative variable derived from analyzing a patient's electroencephalogram that can be used to tailor hypnotic drug doses to a patient's individual requirements.[91] The bispectral index can be used effectively in patient groups that are at particularly high risk for oversedation and hypoxemia, like the elderly and patients with abnormal pulmonary function.[92]

Managing Adverse Effects

During the training process, trainees need to learn the important sedation-related adverse effects and how to manage them correctly. Trainees should be aware of the rescue techniques for each of the commonly encountered adverse effects (**Table 4**). Transient hypoxemia and hypotension represent the most common problems that occur during endoscopic sedation, occurring in 5% to 10% of patients.[24,68,78,93] Serious cardiovascular complications such as myocardial infarction are rare and occur in less than 0.5% of patients.[94]

Upper airway problems requiring basic airway modification maneuvers (eg, chin lift, mask ventilation, nasal airway) are frequent. Cote and colleagues[78] showed in a cohort of 799 patients that 14.4% of patients undergoing endoscopy required some sort of airway modification. Thus, it is recommended that endoscopists should be trained in airway support techniques like jaw-thrust, chin-life, and bag-valve-mask ventilation.[17] It is universally recommended that endoscopists who perform sedation be trained in Basic Life Support skills, which includes bag-valve-mask ventilation and the MSCGE recommend that endoscopists be trained Advanced Cardiac Life Support.[1,2] Although mastery of endotracheal intubation is outside the scope of gastroenterology, airway management training on models and an understanding of how to perform airway rescue maneuvers is a goal of the MSCGE.[1]

The combination of multiple sedative medications increases the risk of respiratory failure by causing synergistic respiratory depression.[95] For patients undergoing moderate sedation who develop severe hypoventilation, pharmacologic reversal agents may be administered (see **Table 3**). Flumazenil abrogates the effects of benzodiazepines by competitively binding to the central nervous system benzodiazepine receptor.[27] Opiates' effects may be reversed by administration of naloxone, which binds competitively to the μ-opioid receptor.[28] However, rapid administration of flumazenil may induce seizures and the use of naloxone in chronic opiate users can induce withdrawal symptoms. Simulators that model hypoventilation during moderate sedation have been used effectively to teach optimal management strategies.[96] Trainees should also be aware of the existence of propofol infusion syndrome, a serious complication event that may result in cardiovascular compromise, metabolic acidic acidosis, rhabdomyolysis, and renal failure.[97]

Table 4 Adverse effects associated with sedation	
	Counter Measure
Hypoxemia	Stop infusion of sedatives
	Increase oxygen supplementation
	Maintain airway
	Jaw-thrust maneuver
	Suctioning
	Mask ventilation
	Nasal airway
	Endotracheal intubation
	Advanced Cardiac Life Support
Hypotension	Electrolyte solution
	Catecholamine infusion
Bradycardia	Atropine

Adapted from American Association for Study of Liver Diseases, American College of Gastroenterology, American Gastroenterological Association Institute, et al. Multisociety sedation curriculum for gastrointestinal endoscopy. Gastrointest Endosc 2012;76:e1–25; and Lee TH, Lee CK. Endoscopic sedation: from training to performance. Clin Endosc 2014;47:141–50.

TRAINING IN POSTSEDATION CARE

The final step of the training process is learning the critical elements of postsedation monitoring and requirements for safe discharge. The intraprocedural monitoring tools (eg, pulse oximetry, blood pressure) are continued in the immediate postprocedure period. Depth of sedation scales (eg, the Observer's Assessment of Alertness/Sedation) can continue to be applied during this period as well. The trainee must be aware of the duration of action of the medications that were given (see **Table 3**). Serious adverse effects of sedation may occur up to 30 minutes after administration of certain medications.[98] Patients who were previously deemed at high cardiopulmonary risk during the preprocedure assessment should continue to be monitored more frequently and possibly for a longer duration after the procedure.

Trainees should understand and apply standardized criteria to assess for recovery from sedation to facilitate a safe and efficient discharge.[17,98,99] The 2 most widely used discharge criteria most used today are the Postanesthetic Discharge Scoring System and the Aldrete scoring system (**Box 1**).[99–102] Trainees should be aware that, even if a patient meets standardized discharge criteria, significant psychomotor delay still exists and specific instructions should be given before discharge in a verbal

---

Box 1
Aldrete score

Respiration

2 = Able to breathe deeply and cough freely

1 = Dyspnea or limited breathing

0 = Apneic

Oxygen saturation

2 = Maintains greater than 92% on room air

1 = Needs O_2 inhalation to maintain O_2 saturation greater than 90%

0 = O_2 saturation less than 90% even with supplemental O_2

Consciousness

2 = Fully awake

1 = Arousable on calling

0 = Not responding

Circulation

2 = BP $\pm$ 20% mm Hg of preanesthetic level

1 = BP $\pm$ 20% to 50% mm Hg of preanesthetic level

0 = BP $\pm$ 50% mm Hg of preanesthetic level

Activity

2 = Able to move 4 extremities

1 = Able to move 2 extremities

0 = Unable to move extremities

Total score = 10. Patients with a score $\geq$8 is fit for discharge.
Abbreviation: BP, blood pressure.
Adapted from Aldrete JA. The post-anesthesia recovery score revisited. J Clin Anesth 1995;7:89; with permission.

and written form. These instructions should include refraining from driving, operating heavy machinery, or engaging in legally binding decisions for 12 to 24 hours.[24,103] After a training program based on the S3 sedation guidelines, the use of formal criterion for discharge after sedation doubled.[46]

ASSESSMENT OF COMPETENCY

Assessment of the trainee's competency is a requirement before independent practice. There are several ways to gauge competency in sedation. One approach to assessing competency is the instructor's observation and critique of a trainee during real procedures. However, this approach to assessing competency may be subjective and unreliable.[104] The major guidelines endorse a more standardized approach using objective examinations of knowledge and web-based teaching modules, in addition to simulation and direct observation.[1,17,23,25,26] Medical record audits and adverse events monitoring can be used to identify incompetency through quality improvement initiatives. Periodic morbidity and mortality conferences to review adverse events can also be used for this purpose.[20]

The European curriculum has been used to develop a number of regional and institutional courses. The European Curriculum's competency assessment evaluates for proficiency in preprocedure assessment, intraproedure and postprocedure care, management of complications, and legal issues.[23] The European competency assessment is done via a formative and summative assessment. The formative assessment includes a review of the trainee's documentation of 30 sedation cases performed during the mentorship period. The summative assessment includes direct observation, debriefing/analytical reflection, and a written examination. Three independent supervisors should take full responsibility for the final summative competency assessment. After successful completion of the curriculum and passing a final examination, trainees receive a competency certificate.[23] Currently, this is awarded by the institution or regional organization sponsoring the course, the eventual goal is for this to be given by the European Society of Gastrointestinal Endoscopy–European Society of and Gastroenterology and Endoscopy Nurses and Associates.[23]

The MSCGE curriculum defines competency to include medical knowledge of pharmacology, airway management, and periprocedural assessment, and recommends testing with objective examinations.[1] However, it also emphasizes proficiency with the informed consent process, practice-based learning, and systems-based practice. It suggests that medical record audits, multisource feedback from staff, and surveys of patient satisfaction may be helpful to measure these competencies. The MSCGE does not offer specific criterion for certification. In most American centers, an institution-specific written or computerized quiz and a certain number of observed cases are required before the granting of moderate sedation privileges.[31] The MSCGE does recommend that specific question on the topics of sedation pharmacology, preprocedure risk stratification (including management of pregnant and lactating women), intraprocedure monitoring, and recovery assessment be included on the American Board of Internal Medicine Gastroenterology Certification Exam. It also recommends that trainees and staff endoscopists maintain Advanced Cardiac Life Support certification.[1]

Although the major consortiums have proposed goals for competency, there is a lack of formal testing mechanisms and studies of their validity.[1,23,25,105] Procedural assessment forms developed by the American Society for Gastrointestinal Endoscopy, which include grading of procedural sedation capabilities, are often used in fellowship programs to gauge competency, but have not been fully validated.[20,106] A performance assessment tool has been developed to assess proficiency of nurses training in propofol sedation.[105] Jensen and colleagues[105] proposed a 17-item nurse-administered propofol assessment tool to provide proficiency evaluation for endoscopy nurses who underwent a structured curriculum on propofol sedation. They validated this assessment tool in a simulation setting with video-based assessments done by 3 experts. Nurses who had completed a structured curriculum in sedation scored significantly higher than novices on the nurse-administered propofol assessment tool and there was favorable interrater reliability.[105] Although validated testing mechanisms for training endoscopists have not been developed, future studies on the subject may benefit from incorporating procedure assessment surveys from both the operator and the patient into the testing to provide a clinically meaningful evaluation of procedure sedation quality.[107] After assessing for competency, formal proficiency feedback or debriefing should be given to improve trainee satisfaction, learning, and perceptions of sedation principles.[108]

Trainees should realize that, even after undergoing a full training process and certification, certain skills continue to improve with additional clinical experiences. Schulz and colleagues[109] showed that inexperienced anesthesia providers spent more time on monitoring tasks versus manual tasks during critical incidents compared with experienced providers. These findings indicate that more experienced sedation providers are able to interpret data more quickly and are able to use their time more efficiently for interventional tasks.[109] Multiple large series have demonstrated that the incidence of adverse events during sedation for endoscopy decreases as provider experience grows.[9,61,110]

Role of Simulation in Competency Assessment

Simulation is a mechanism to both teach endoscopists sedation techniques and test trainees for competency. In the field of aviation, it has been demonstrated to decrease the incidence of human error.[96] Although their use is much more established in anesthesiology training, simulation has recently been integrated into gastrointestinal endoscopy training.[18] Simulation-based training involves creating specific case scenarios in a controlled and realistic environment with standard equipment that requires the trainee and teams to perform routine and emergent interventions.[111–116] The trainee is given the unique opportunity of being able to practice endoscopic sedation without the fear of making catastrophic errors.[18] They also allow for the trainees to gain hands-on experience managing adverse events such as arrhythmias and drug reactions that are relatively rare in clinical practice. The European curriculum and MSCGE currently recommends having full-scale patient simulator training as part of the training process.[1,23,24]

Several studies have demonstrated the effectiveness of simulation training in endoscopic sedation. Kiesslich and colleagues[96] used a combined full-scale patient simulator and endoscopy simulator in a crisis management workshop to improve significantly the endoscopic performance of a hundred endoscopists who already had greater than 1 year of endoscopy experience. Westfelt and colleagues[117] developed simulations of 4 clinical scenarios to successfully teach endoscopists and endoscopy nurses the typical sedation side effects of propofol. Levine and colleagues[118] showed that endoscopists' sedation knowledge and clinical skills, as evaluated by pretraining and posttraining testing, can be increased by the implementation of full-scale, high-fidelity simulation training. Simulation training may also benefit patient safety by reinforcing sedation standards. A study on a simulation-based sedation training course developed in Japan showed that the training course was able to significantly improve endoscopist attitudes toward multiple safety measures that were derived from guidelines.[119]

Simulation-based competency assessments offers several benefits such as allowing for a collective assessment of the endoscopist working in tandem with the entire team rather than just the individual endoscopist and a combined evaluation of technical performance (eg, vital sign monitoring), behavioral performance (eg, decision making), and ethical decision making of trainees in rare adverse scenarios.[112–116,120] It has also been used to reliably gauge the acquisition of new sedation skills such as management of overdose and administration of new sedative agents.[117] However, simulator-based tests are a challenge to create because they need to be constructed with reliability and validity measurements, rater training, and multiple occasions of testing and piloting scenarios.[121] Additionally, sedation simulation training is limited at many institutions because of the requirements for an anesthesia instructor, simulation technician, and the high cost of simulation equipment.[18]

SUMMARY

Sedation improves the comfort and quality of endoscopy, but requires training and experience. Endoscopic trainees need to be competent in the performance of preprocedure workup, including patient evaluation and consent, intraprocedure management including drug administration, and postprocedure requirements including monitoring and safe discharge. The establishment of training curricula by the American, European, and other societies has led to a more consistent approach to teaching sedation. Simulators hold promise as a method to systematically teach sedation practices. Nevertheless, formal training courses are not widely available and there are no validated methods to test competence. Future controlled studies and initiatives are needed to develop a systematic approach for the training of endoscopic sedation and to develop high-fidelity methods to measure theoretical and technical competence.

REFERENCES

1. American Association for Study of Liver Diseases, American College of Gastroenterology, American Gastroenterological Association Institute, et al. Multisociety sedation curriculum for gastrointestinal endoscopy. Gastrointest Endosc 2012;76:e1–25.
2. American Society of Anesthesiologists Task Force on Sedation and Analgesia by Non-Anesthesiologists. Practice guidelines for sedation and analgesia by non-anesthesiologists. Anesthesiology 2002;96:1004–17.
3. Khiani VS, Soulos P, Gancayco J, et al. Anesthesiologist involvement in screening colonoscopy: temporal trends and cost implications in the Medicare population. Clin Gastroenterol Hepatol 2012;10:58–64.e1.
4. Hassan NE, Betz BW, Cole MR, et al. Randomized controlled trial for intermittent versus continuous propofol sedation for pediatric brain and spine magnetic resonance imaging studies. Pediatr Crit Care Med 2011;12:e262–5.
5. Dumonceau JM. Nonanesthesiologist administration of propofol: it's all about money. Endoscopy 2012;44:453–5.
6. Sieg A, bng-Study-Group, Beck S, et al. Safety analysis of endoscopist-directed propofol sedation: a prospective, national multicenter study of 24 441 patients in German outpatient practices. J Gastroenterol Hepatol 2014;29:517–23.
7. Frieling T, Heise J, Kreysel C, et al. Sedation-associated complications in endoscopy–prospective multicentre survey of 191142 patients. Z Gastroenterol 2013; 51:568–72.

8. Goudra BG, Singh PM, Gouda G, et al. Safety of Non-anesthesia Provider-Administered Propofol (NAAP) sedation in advanced gastrointestinal endoscopic procedures: comparative meta-analysis of pooled results. Dig Dis Sci 2015;60: 2612–27.

9. Rex DK, Heuss LT, Walker JA, et al. Trained registered nurses/endoscopy teams can administer propofol safely for endoscopy. Gastroenterology 2005;129: 1384–91.

10. Rex DK, Deenadayalu VP, Eid E, et al. Endoscopist-directed administration of propofol: a worldwide safety experience. Gastroenterology 2009;137:1229–37 [quiz: 1518–9].

11. Kulling D, Orlandi M, Inauen W. Propofol sedation during endoscopic procedures: how much staff and monitoring are necessary? Gastrointest Endosc 2007;66:443–9.

12. Burtea DE, Dimitriu A, Malos AE, et al. Current role of non-anesthesiologist administered propofol sedation in advanced interventional endoscopy. World J Gastrointest Endosc 2015;7:981–6.

13. Horiuchi A, Nakayama Y, Hidaka N, et al. Low-dose propofol sedation for diagnostic esophagogastroduodenoscopy: results in 10,662 adults. Am J Gastroenterol 2009;104:1650–5.

14. Perel A. Non-anaesthesiologists should not be allowed to administer propofol for procedural sedation: a consensus statement of 21 European national societies of anaesthesia. Eur J Anaesthesiol 2011;28:580–4.

15. American Society of Anesthesiologists. Statement on granting privileges to nonanesthesiologist physicians for personally administering or supervising deep sedation. 2012. Available at: http://www.asahq.org/~/media/sites/asahq/files/public/resources/standards-guidelines/statement-on-granting-privileges-to-nonanesthesiologist-administering-physicians-deep-sedation.pdf.

16. Petrini J, Egan JV. Risk management regarding sedation/analgesia. Gastrointest Endosc Clin N Am 2004;14:401–14.

17. Cohen LB, Delegge MH, Aisenberg J, et al. AGA Institute review of endoscopic sedation. Gastroenterology 2007;133:675–701.

18. DeMaria S Jr, Levine AI, Cohen LB. Human patient simulation and its role in endoscopic sedation training. Gastrointest Endosc Clin N Am 2008;18:801–13.

19. Tse T, Armstrong D, Barkun AN. Training in gastrointestinal endoscopy in Canada: a survey of program directors in gastroenterology. Gastrointest Endosc 2004;59:P123.

20. Training Committee of the American Society for Gastrointestinal Endoscopy, Vargo JJ, Ahmad AS, et al. Training in patient monitoring and sedation and analgesia. Gastrointest Endosc 2007;66:7–10.

21. Dumonceau JM, Andriulli A, Deviere J, et al. European Society of Gastrointestinal Endoscopy (ESGE) guideline: prophylaxis of post-ERCP pancreatitis. Endoscopy 2010;42:503–15.

22. Riphaus A, Bitter H. Short version S3 guideline sedation for gastrointestinal endoscopy und medicolegal implications. Z Gastroenterol 2012;50:407–10.

23. Dumonceau JM, Riphaus A, Beilenhoff U, et al. European curriculum for sedation training in gastrointestinal endoscopy: position statement of the European Society of Gastrointestinal Endoscopy (ESGE) and European Society of Gastroenterology and Endoscopy Nurses and Associates (ESGENA). Endoscopy 2013;45:496–504.

24. Dumonceau JM, Riphaus A, Schreiber F, et al. Non-anesthesiologist administration of propofol for gastrointestinal endoscopy: European Society of

Gastrointestinal Endoscopy, European Society of Gastroenterology and Endoscopy Nurses and Associates Guideline–Updated June 2015. Endoscopy 2015; 47:1175–89.

25. Igea F, Casellas JA, Gonzalez-Huix F, et al. Sedation for gastrointestinal endoscopy. Endoscopy 2014;46:720–31.

26. Riphaus A, Wehrmann T, Weber B, et al. S3-guidelines–sedation in gastrointestinal endoscopy. Z Gastroenterol 2008;46:1298–330.

27. Obara K, Haruma K, Irisawa A, et al. Guidelines for sedation in gastroenterological endoscopy. Dig Endosc 2015;27:435–49.

28. Thomson A, Andrew G, Jones DB. Optimal sedation for gastrointestinal endoscopy: review and recommendations. J Gastroenterol Hepatol 2010;25:469–78.

29. Behrens A, Kainzinger FA, Nolling T, et al. S3 guideline on "sedation in gastrointestinal endoscopy": how much does the new guideline cost in everyday hospital work? A calculation model and analysis of implementation in 2011 among ALGK members. Z Gastroenterol 2012;50:1002–7 [in German].

30. Kang SH, Hyun JJ. Preparation and patient evaluation for safe gastrointestinal endoscopy. Clin Endosc 2013;46:212–8.

31. Berzin TM. Endoscopic sedation training in gastroenterology fellowship. Gastrointest Endosc 2010;71:597–9.

32. Cohen LB. Inspire or expire: the safety of endoscopic sedation in patients with sleep apnea. Gastrointest Endosc 2014;79:445–7.

33. Cha JM, Jeun JW, Pack KM, et al. Risk of sedation for diagnostic esophagogastroduodenoscopy in obstructive sleep apnea patients. World J Gastroenterol 2013;19:4745–51.

34. Wani S, Azar R, Hovis CE, et al. Obesity as a risk factor for sedation-related complications during propofol-mediated sedation for advanced endoscopic procedures. Gastrointest Endosc 2011;74:1238–47.

35. Vargo JJ. Procedural sedation and obesity: waters left uncharted. Gastrointest Endosc 2009;70:980–4.

36. Langeron O, Masso E, Huraux C, et al. Prediction of difficult mask ventilation. Anesthesiology 2000;92:1229–36.

37. Silvis SE, Nebel O, Rogers G, et al. Endoscopic complications. Results of the 1974 American Society for Gastrointestinal Endoscopy Survey. JAMA 1976; 235:928–30.

38. Louis S, Bassett M, Clarke A, et al. Anaesthetic support for endoscopic retrograde cholangiopancreatograms in Australian teaching hospitals. Intern Med J 2004;34:368–9.

39. Dripps RD, Lamont A, Eckenhoff JE. The role of anesthesia in surgical mortality. JAMA 1961;178:261–6.

40. Zakeri N, Coda S, Webster S, et al. Risk factors for endoscopic sedation reversal events: a five-year retrospective study. Frontline Gastroenterol 2015;6:270–7.

41. Sharma VK, Nguyen CC, Crowell MD, et al. A national study of cardiopulmonary unplanned events after GI endoscopy. Gastrointest Endosc 2007;66:27–34.

42. Heuss LT, Schnieper P, Drewe J, et al. Safety of propofol for conscious sedation during endoscopic procedures in high-risk patients-a prospective, controlled study. Am J Gastroenterol 2003;98:1751–7.

43. Dietrich CG, Kottmann T, Diedrich A, et al. Sedation-associated complications in endoscopy are not reduced significantly by implementation of the German S-3-guideline and occur in a severe manner only in patients with ASA class III and higher. Scand J Gastroenterol 2013;48:1082–7.

44. Ooi M, Thomson A. Morbidity and mortality of endoscopist-directed nurse-administered propofol sedation (EDNAPS) in a tertiary referral center. Endosc Int Open 2015;3:E393–7.

45. Cohen LB, Ladas SD, Vargo JJ, et al. Sedation in digestive endoscopy: the Athens international position statements. Aliment Pharmacol Ther 2010;32: 425–42.

46. Schilling D, Leicht K, Beilenhoff U, et al. Impact of S3 training courses "Sedation and Emergency Management in Endoscopy for Endoscopy Nurses and Assisting Personnel" on the process and structure quality in gastroenterological endoscopy in practices and clinics - results of a nationwide survey. Z Gastroenterol 2013;51: 619–27.

47. Qureshi WA, Zuckerman MJ, Adler DG, et al. ASGE guideline: modifications in endoscopic practice for the elderly. Gastrointest Endosc 2006;63:566–9.

48. Peacock JE, Lewis RP, Reilly CS, et al. Effect of different rates of infusion of propofol for induction of anaesthesia in elderly patients. Br J Anaesth 1990; 65:346–52.

49. Darling E. Practical considerations in sedating the elderly. Crit Care Nurs Clin North Am 1997;9:371–80.

50. Cotton PB. Analysis of 59 ERCP lawsuits; mainly about indications. Gastrointest Endosc 2006;63:378–82 [quiz: 464].

51. Quine MA, Bell GD, McCloy RF, et al. Prospective audit of upper gastrointestinal endoscopy in two regions of England: safety, staffing, and sedation methods. Gut 1995;36:462–7.

52. Feld AD. Endoscopic sedation: medicolegal considerations. Gastrointest Endosc Clin N Am 2008;18:783–8.

53. Berg JW, Apfelbaum PS, Grisso T. Constructing competence: formulating standards of legal competence to make medical decisions. Rutgers Law Rev 1996;48:345–71.

54. Feld AD. Informed consent: not just for procedures anymore. Am J Gastroenterol 2004;99:977–80.

55. Training Committee. American Society for Gastrointestinal Endoscopy. Training guideline for use of propofol in gastrointestinal endoscopy. Gastrointest Endosc 2004;60:167–72.

56. Ely EW, Truman B, Shintani A, et al. Monitoring sedation status over time in ICU patients: reliability and validity of the Richmond Agitation-Sedation Scale (RASS). JAMA 2003;289:2983–91.

57. Ramsay MA, Savege TM, Simpson BR, et al. Controlled sedation with alphax-alone-alphadolone. Br Med J 1974;2:656–9.

58. Riker RR, Picard JT, Fraser GL. Prospective evaluation of the sedation-agitation Scale for adult critically ill patients. Crit Care Med 1999;27:1325–9.

59. Chernik DA, Gillings D, Laine H, et al. Validity and reliability of the observer's assessment of alertness/sedation scale: study with intravenous midazolam. J Clin Psychopharmacol 1990;10:244–51.

60. Chawla S, Katz A, Attar BM, et al. Endoscopic retrograde cholangiopancreatography under moderate sedation and factors predicting need for anesthesiologist directed sedation: a county hospital experience. World J Gastrointest Endosc 2013;5:160–4.

61. Jensen JT, Vilmann P, Horsted T, et al. Nurse-administered propofol sedation for endoscopy: a risk analysis during an implementation phase. Endoscopy 2011; 43:716–22.

62. Group Gee. Evaluation of conscious sedation for endoscopy in Germany. Gastrointest Endosc 2000;51:AB295.
63. Cohen LB, Wecsler JS, Gaetano JN, et al. Endoscopic sedation in the United States: results from a nationwide survey. Am J Gastroenterol 2006;101:967–74.
64. Allonen H, Ziegler G, Klotz U. Midazolam kinetics. Clin Pharmacol Ther 1981;30: 653–61.
65. Zakko SF, Seifert HA, Gross JB. A comparison of midazolam and diazepam for conscious sedation during colonoscopy in a prospective double-blind study. Gastrointest Endosc 1999;49:684–9.
66. Bailey PL, Pace NL, Ashburn MA, et al. Frequent hypoxemia and apnea after sedation with midazolam and fentanyl. Anesthesiology 1990;73:826–30.
67. Macken E, Gevers AM, Hendrickx A, et al. Midazolam versus diazepam in lipid emulsion as conscious sedation for colonoscopy with or without reversal of sedation with flumazenil. Gastrointest Endosc 1998;47:57–61.
68. McQuaid KR, Laine L. A systematic review and meta-analysis of randomized, controlled trials of moderate sedation for routine endoscopic procedures. Gastrointest Endosc 2008;67:910–23.
69. Papachristou GI, Gleeson FC, Papachristou DJ, et al. Endoscopist administered sedation during ERCP: impact of chronic narcotic/benzodiazepine use and predictive risk of reversal agent utilization. Am J Gastroenterol 2007;102: 738–43.
70. Tu RH, Grewall P, Leung JW, et al. Diphenhydramine as an adjunct to sedation for colonoscopy: a double-blind randomized, placebo-controlled study. Gastrointest Endosc 2006;63:87–94.
71. Varadarajulu S, Eloubeidi MA, Tamhane A, et al. Prospective randomized trial evaluating ketamine for advanced endoscopic procedures in difficult to sedate patients. Aliment Pharmacol Ther 2007;25:987–97.
72. Habib AS, Gan TJ. The use of droperidol before and after the Food and Drug Administration black box warning: a survey of the members of the Society of ambulatory anesthesia. J Clin Anesth 2008;20:35–9.
73. Cohen LB. Making 1+1=3: improving sedation through drug synergy. Gastrointest Endosc 2011;73:215–7.
74. Vargo JJ, Zuccaro G Jr, Dumot JA, et al. Gastroenterologist-administered propofol versus meperidine and midazolam for advanced upper endoscopy: a prospective, randomized trial. Gastroenterology 2002;123:8–16.
75. Levitzky BE, Lopez R, Dumot JA, et al. Moderate sedation for elective upper endoscopy with balanced propofol versus fentanyl and midazolam alone: a randomized clinical trial. Endoscopy 2012;44:13–20.
76. Dewitt J, McGreevy K, Sherman S, et al. Nurse-administered propofol sedation compared with midazolam and meperidine for EUS: a prospective, randomized trial. Gastrointest Endosc 2008;68:499–509.
77. Berzin TM, Sanaka S, Barnett SR, et al. A prospective assessment of sedation-related adverse events and patient and endoscopist satisfaction in ERCP with anesthesiologist-administered sedation. Gastrointest Endosc 2011;73:710–7.
78. Cote GA, Hovis RM, Ansstas MA, et al. Incidence of sedation-related complications with propofol use during advanced endoscopic procedures. Clin Gastroenterol Hepatol 2010;8:137–42.
79. Inadomi JM, Gunnarsson CL, Rizzo JA, et al. Projected increased growth rate of anesthesia professional-delivered sedation for colonoscopy and EGD in the United States: 2009 to 2015. Gastrointest Endosc 2010;72:580–6.

80. Liu H, Waxman DA, Main R, et al. Utilization of anesthesia services during outpatient endoscopies and colonoscopies and associated spending in 2003-2009. JAMA 2012;307:1178–84.
81. Heuss LT, Froehlich F, Beglinger C. Nonanesthesiologist-administered propofol sedation: from the exception to standard practice. Sedation and monitoring trends over 20 years. Endoscopy 2012;44:504–11.
82. Crantock L, Cowen AE, Ward M, et al. Supplemental low flow oxygen prevents hypoxia during endoscopic cholangiopancreatography. Gastrointest Endosc 1992;38:418–20.
83. Bell GD, Bown S, Morden A, et al. Prevention of hypoxaemia during upper-gastrointestinal endoscopy by means of oxygen via nasal cannulae. Lancet 1987;1:1022–4.
84. Bowling TE, Hadjiminas CL, Polson RJ, et al. Effects of supplemental oxygen on cardiac rhythm during upper gastrointestinal endoscopy: a randomised controlled double blind trial. Gut 1993;34:1492–7.
85. Bell GD, Quine A, Antrobus JH, et al. Upper gastrointestinal endoscopy: a prospective randomized study comparing continuous supplemental oxygen via the nasal or oral route. Gastrointest Endosc 1992;38:319–25.
86. Riphaus A, Geist F, Wehrmann T. Endoscopic sedation and monitoring practice in Germany: re-evaluation from the first nationwide survey 3 years after the implementation of an evidence and consent based national guideline. Z Gastroenterol 2013;51:1082–8.
87. Lightdale JR, Goldmann DA, Feldman HA, et al. Microstream capnography improves patient monitoring during moderate sedation: a randomized, controlled trial. Pediatrics 2006;117:e1170–8.
88. Vargo JJ, Zuccaro G Jr, Dumot JA, et al. Automated graphic assessment of respiratory activity is superior to pulse oximetry and visual assessment for the detection of early respiratory depression during therapeutic upper endoscopy. Gastrointest Endosc 2002;55:826–31.
89. Qadeer MA, Vargo JJ, Dumot JA, et al. Capnographic monitoring of respiratory activity improves safety of sedation for endoscopic cholangiopancreatography and ultrasonography. Gastroenterology 2009;136:1568–76 [quiz: 1819–20].
90. Carlisle H. Promoting the use of capnography in acute care settings: an evidence-based practice project. J Perianesth Nurs 2015;30:201–8.
91. Johansen JW. Update on bispectral index monitoring. Best Pract Res Clin Anaesthesiol 2006;20:81–99.
92. Gotoda T, Okada H, Hori K, et al. Propofol sedation with a target-controlled infusion pump and bispectral index monitoring system in elderly patients during a complex upper endoscopy procedure. Gastrointest Endosc 2015;83(4):756–64.
93. Lee TH, Lee CK. Endoscopic sedation: from training to performance. Clin Endosc 2014;47:141–50.
94. Gangi S, Saidi F, Patel K, et al. Cardiovascular complications after GI endoscopy: occurrence and risks in a large hospital system. Gastrointest Endosc 2004;60:679–85.
95. Arrowsmith JB, Gerstman BB, Fleischer DE, et al. Results from the American Society for Gastrointestinal Endoscopy/U.S. Food and Drug Administration collaborative study on complication rates and drug use during gastrointestinal endoscopy. Gastrointest Endosc 1991;37:421–7.
96. Kiesslich R, Moenk S, Reinhardt K, et al. Combined simulation training: a new concept and workshop is useful for crisis management in gastrointestinal endoscopy. Z Gastroenterol 2005;43:1031–9.

97. Riker RR, Glisic EK, Fraser GL. Propofol infusion syndrome: difficult to recognize, difficult to study. Crit Care Med 2009;37:3169–70.

98. Newman DH, Azer MM, Pitetti RD, et al. When is a patient safe for discharge after procedural sedation? The timing of adverse effect events in 1367 pediatric procedural sedations. Ann Emerg Med 2003;42:627–35.

99. Chung F, Chan VW, Ong D. A post-anesthetic discharge scoring system for home readiness after ambulatory surgery. J Clin Anesth 1995;7:500–6.

100. Aldrete JA, Kroulik D. A postanesthetic recovery score. Anesth Analg 1970;49: 924–34.

101. Aldrete JA. The post-anesthesia recovery score revisited. J Clin Anesth 1995;7: 89–91.

102. Amornyotin S, Chalayonnavin W, Kongphlay S. Recovery pattern and home-readiness after ambulatory gastrointestinal endoscopy. J Med Assoc Thai 2007;90:2352–8.

103. Willey J, Vargo JJ, Connor JT, et al. Quantitative assessment of psychomotor recovery after sedation and analgesia for outpatient EGD. Gastrointest Endosc 2002;56:810–6.

104. Moorthy K, Munz Y, Sarker SK, et al. Objective assessment of technical skills in surgery. BMJ 2003;327:1032–7.

105. Jensen JT, Konge L, Moller A, et al. Endoscopy nurse-administered propofol sedation performance. Development of an assessment tool and a reliability testing model. Scand J Gastroenterol 2014;49:1014–9.

106. Committee AT, Sedlack RE, Coyle WJ, et al. ASGE's assessment of competency in endoscopy evaluation tools for colonoscopy and EGD. Gastrointest Endosc 2014;79:1–7.

107. Leffler DA, Bukoye B, Sawhney M, et al. Development and validation of the PROcedural Sedation Assessment Survey (PROSAS) for assessment of procedural sedation quality. Gastrointest Endosc 2015;81:194–203.e1.

108. Komasawa N, Sanuki T, Fujiwara S, et al. Significance of debriefing methods in simulation-based sedation training courses for medical safety improvement in Japan. Springerplus 2014;3:637.

109. Schulz CM, Schneider E, Fritz L, et al. Visual attention of anaesthetists during simulated critical incidents. Br J Anaesth 2011;106:807–13.

110. Heuss LT, Schnieper P, Drewe J, et al. Risk stratification and safe administration of propofol by registered nurses supervised by the gastroenterologist: a prospective observational study of more than 2000 cases. Gastrointest Endosc 2003;57:664–71.

111. Gaba DM, DeAnda A. A comprehensive anesthesia simulation environment: recreating the operating room for research and training. Anesthesiology 1988;69: 387–94.

112. Meurling L, Hedman L, Sandahl C, et al. Systematic simulation-based team training in a Swedish intensive care unit: a diverse response among critical care professions. BMJ Qual Saf 2013;22:485–94.

113. Wallin CJ, Meurling L, Hedman L, et al. Target-focused medical emergency team training using a human patient simulator: effects on behaviour and attitude. Med Educ 2007;41:173–80.

114. Kobayashi L, Dunbar-Viveiros JA, Devine J, et al. Pilot-phase findings from high-fidelity In Situ medical simulation investigation of emergency department procedural sedation. Simul Healthc 2012;7:81–94.

115. Desilets DJ, Banerjee S, Barth BA, et al. Endoscopic simulators. Gastrointest Endosc 2011;73:861–7.

116. Gaba DM, Howard SK, Flanagan B, et al. Assessment of clinical performance during simulated crises using both technical and behavioral ratings. Anesthesiology 1998;89:8–18.
117. Westfelt P, Hedman L, Axelsson Lindkvist M, et al. Training nonanesthetist administration of propofol for gastrointestinal endoscopy in scenario-based full-scale hybrid simulation–a pilot study. Scand J Gastroenterol 2013;48:1354–8.
118. Levine AI, Sanyal S, Dikman AE, et al. Moderate sedation training using high-fidelity simulation. Gastrointest Endosc 2008;67:AB301.
119. Komasawa N, Fujiwara S, Atagi K, et al. Effects of a simulation-based sedation training course on non-anesthesiologists' attitudes toward sedation and analgesia. J Anesth 2014;28:785–9.
120. Hodges B. Assessment in the post-psychometric era: learning to love the subjective and collective. Med Teach 2013;35:564–8.
121. Edler AA, Fanning RG, Chen MI, et al. Patient simulation: a literary synthesis of assessment tools in anesthesiology. J Educ Eval Health Prof 2009;6:3.
122. Hillman DR, Walsh JH, Maddison KJ, et al. Evolution of changes in upper airway collapsibility during slow induction of anesthesia with propofol. Anesthesiology 2009;111:63–71.

Endoscopic Sedation
Medicolegal Considerations

Andreas A. Kralios, JD, Kayla A. Feld, JD, Andrew D. Feld, MD, JD*

KEYWORDS

- Informed consent • Endoscopy • Medicolegal risk • Malpractice

KEY POINTS

- Informed consent for endoscopy should include discussion of the risks, benefits, and alternatives in sedation, thus including informed consent for sedation.
- The endoscopist should be aware of the possibility that a patient whose sedation is not felt to be sufficient from the patient's perspective may withdraw consent for the procedure.
- The endoscopist should keep up to date regarding the standards of care for monitoring sedation, and for choosing anesthesiologist/anesthetist sedation for appropriate patients.

MALPRACTICE LAW REVIEW

Consider a brief review of malpractice concepts to guide our understanding of the legal aspects of sedation.[1]

Risk Management

Risk management programs attempt to understand actual risk by an analysis of malpractice data, and use that analysis to develop awareness of specific risks in specific treatment encounters. Thus, the goal of risk management programs is to develop preventive measures to reduce both patient injury and malpractice risk.

Tort of Negligence

A malpractice action against a physician typically takes form in the tort of negligence, a "civil wrong." The plaintiff's attorney must prove 4 elements: (1) that the physician has an obligation (duty) of care for that individual, (2) that the duty was violated (breach) by practice below the applicable standard of care, (3) that substandard practice caused the harm asserted (causation), and (4) that the plaintiff suffers cognizable and compensable harm (damages).

Disclaimer: These are general thoughts presented for their educational value, and are NOT intended to represent specific legal advice. That would require independent legal counsel.
This is a revised version of an article appearing in volume 18, number 4, October 2008, of *Gastrointestinal Endoscopy Clinics of North America*.
University of Washington, Seattle, WA, USA
* Corresponding author.
E-mail address: afeld@u.washington.edu

Standard of Care

Guidelines

Establishing that the provider has violated the standard of care is often the most critical element of the lawsuit. Expert witness testimony is usually required to explain the current standard of care and how the provider has practiced below it. However, expert witnesses are not needed under the so-called common knowledge[2] or obvious occurrence[3] exception, wherein the wrong committed is within the realm of a layperson's comprehension (eg, a sponge retained in the abdomen at surgery or amputation of the wrong limb). In addition, expert witnesses are unnecessary under a similar but technically separate doctrine called *res ipsa loquitur* (the thing speaks for itself), a legal term applying to a narrow category of malpractice cases in which the jury may infer negligence from the mere fact of an accident's occurrence.[4] Whereas some jurisdictions openly disfavor application of *res ipsa loquitur* in medical malpractice cases,[5] other jurisdictions apply it in common knowledge/obvious occurrence cases.[6] Furthermore, with increasing frequency, respected national guidelines have become a key element used to establish the standard of care. Nonetheless, although a court will regard such guidelines as relevant evidence, it typically will not allow them, standing alone, to establish the standard of care for any given situation.[7]

Informed Consent

Because informed consent requires a communication between provider and patient, and because studies of malpractice risk note that better communication reduces malpractice risk, the process of informed consent can actually be a provider's tool to reduce malpractice risk. Further, the process of disclosing the inherent risks of a procedure essentially asks the patient to accept that risk as part of the performance of the procedure. This transfers the risk of a nonperfect sedation from the endoscopist to the patient, who assumes the risk with the decision to proceed despite the knowledge of sedation and procedural risks. The risk shift does not apply to substandard care, but would apply to many of the known complications of procedures and sedation that may occur even with appropriate technical performance of the procedure.

The patient must be competent to understand the information disclosed. There must be no duress. Material risks should be disclosed. The standard in most jurisdictions is a patient-based standard, not physician-based standard. That means we are obligated to inform based on what a reasonable patient would want to hear (as interpreted/decided by a jury), rather than what a reasonable physician believes should be disclosed.

Material risks

Not every possible risk must be disclosed, only those a reasonable patient would wish to know in make an appropriate, intelligent decision whether or not to submit to surgery or treatment.[8] These have been termed "material risks," and are specific to each procedure and patient situation. There are guiding principles that can be used to help determine what an average patient (and average jury!) would find significant. The 4 elements of risk the physician needs to consider include (1) the nature of the risk, (2) the magnitude of the risk (seriousness), (3) the probability that the risk may occur, and (4) the imminence of the risk.

Vicarious Liability

Vicarious liability is a legal concept that extends liability for a wrongdoing beyond the original wrongdoer to persons who have not committed a wrong, but on whose behalf the wrongdoers acted. The primary practical importance of this concept is that it provides the plaintiff with additional financially responsible defendants who likely have greater resources than the original defendant. Although vicarious liability traditionally arises from employer–employee or other agency relationships, for the practicing physician, the implications of this concept are that physicians can be held legally liable not only for their own actions, but also for the actions of others for whom they have supervisory responsibility. This holds even if the gastroenterologist had neither personally committed, nor even was aware of, the wrongful act. When the negligence of a subordinate is imputed to the gastroenterologist, she or he is said to be vicariously liable. For example, a gastroenterology group that directly employs and supervises a nurse anesthetist as part of their group could be held responsible if that anesthetist negligently reuses syringes.

RISK MANAGEMENT

Because Aisenberg and colleagues[9] and Cohen and coworkers[10] have presented data estimating that sedation probably accounts for 40% to 50% of procedure-related complications, procedural sedation is a topic worthy of our attention. Liability may arise from failure to perform sedation according to the standard of care, or the failure to obtain appropriate informed consent. Further, an endoscopist can be included in a lawsuit both when the endoscopist is responsible for the sedation, and potentially even if an anesthesia provider is instead responsible for the sedation. As procedures have become more complex, and can be performed on very ill patients, the potential for both adverse outcome and negligence increases. Finally, if there are specialty-related political disagreements, adversarial expert witness debates may occur. Thus, endoscopic sedation is an appropriate area of concern for the gastroenterologist to develop risk management strategies.[11,12]

CONSENT ISSUES

Endoscopists are required to disclose necessary information to allow for informed consent by the patient.[13] However, past studies have suggested that although the vast majority of endoscopists have obtained preprocedure consent, many did not routinely discuss sedation as part of the preprocedural consent discussion. Open access endoscopy poses additional problems for sedation consent. A patient may be given blanket reassurance by their primary care provider that they will be totally asleep and experience no discomfort whatsoever. The prudent endoscopist using moderate or conscious sedation may wish to dispel the notion of guaranteed sedation. Some patients, particularly those with antecedent use of narcotics and/or sedatives, may have varying degrees of awareness. There have been scenarios involving upset patients and lawsuits relating to claims of "undersedation" complications.[14]

POSSIBLE WITHDRAWAL OF CONSENT

The conscientious gastroenterologist may be faced with a situation in which, the sedated patient rouses from the conscious sedation haze and says, "Stop!" A British survey demonstrated uncertainty among gastroenterologists over what to do in response.[15] The nature of conscious sedation is such that a patient may perceive, but may not be aware of, the context and surrounding to sufficiently understand the implications of a demand to stop the procedure: a possible lesser procedure without therapeutic capacity, or a repeat colonoscopy after a repeat colon preparation. The discomfort is likely to be short lived and the procedure safe and successful, and often the patient has no recall of difficulty or any request to stop the procedure. Additional medication, along with certain other techniques, allow for more comfortable completion. Indeed, the patient may wish the discomfort to stop, not the procedure!

However, the colonoscopist and staff must be aware that consent can be withdrawn. If a physician were to persist after consent was truly revoked by a competent patient, the physician is then proceeding without consent, and could be accused of battery. Indeed, courts have held that continued treatment after consent has been withdrawn gives rise to a medical battery claim.[16]

In such a scenario, some courts hold that withdrawal of consent may subject providers to liability only if it follows a 2-part test. First, the patient "must act or use language which can be subject to no other inference and which must be unquestioned responses from a clear and rational mind. These actions and utterances of the patient must be such as to leave no room for doubt in the minds of reasonable men that in view of all the circumstances consent was actually withdrawn."[17] Second, if consent is withdrawn, "it must be medically feasible … to desist in the treatment or examination at that point without the cessation being detrimental to the patient's health or life."[17] In other words, under this particular test, withdrawal of consent must be virtually unmistakable, and the provider carrying out a medical procedure must be permitted to discontinue the procedure in a medically safe way.

Nevertheless, consider a patient who has preprocedure chronic use of pain and anxiolytic medications and despite high doses of benzodiazepines and narcotics is not very sedated. This patient may well be alert enough to intend to revoke consent, and remembers office staff holding him down while he is demanding the procedure stop. Now consider that patient describing that scene to a jury. Now consider that patient describing that scene to a jury in a jurisdiction that does not follow the above 2-part test and instead applies a lenient analysis toward withdrawal of consent.

Furthermore, because withdrawal of consent is equal to no consent, providers must know the critical distinction between a lack of "consent" and a lack of "informed consent." Allegations that there was no consent at all are leveled as a battery claim. Meanwhile, allegations of no informed consent mean relevant material risks of treatment or procedure were not disclosed, which touch on the standard of care and thus are brought as negligence.[18] The practical differences for the provider are that (1) battery does not require expert witnesses, (2) punitive damage awards are available under battery, and (3) malpractice insurance frequently will not cover intentional torts like battery.[19]

The senior author surmises, on the basis of conversations with experienced colonoscopists, that most requests to stop are not truly withdrawal of consent, but an artifact of sedation-causing misperception of the context of procedural activity. Nevertheless, the prudent colonoscopist will carefully evaluate a request to stop, to be as certain as possible that it is not a true withdrawal of consent for the procedure, which would mandate withdrawal of the instrument. The colonoscopist may temporarily cease insertion and converse with the patient. This may establish that the patient does in fact wish to proceed or, alternatively, is no longer conscious enough to withdraw consent or otherwise request the procedure stop.[20] On 1 hand, if a very sedated patient rouses briefly to semicoherently mumble "stop," and the physician aborts the procedure, she may have a lot of explaining to do to the unhappy patient who remembers nothing about a request to stop, but a lot about the colonoscopy preparation the patient is now asked to repeat. On the other hand, picture a lightly sedated patient (perhaps coaxed into the examination by a concerned spouse) who experiences difficulty with the procedure, who truly changes his mind about the procedure and repeatedly asserts that the procedure should stop. If the colonoscopist ignores this request, serious consequences could result. There are no easy answers. Listen carefully to the patient, and to the endoscopy nursing staff. If an experienced nursing staff is uncomfortable continuing, this is important information for the colonoscopist. Also, those are the individuals who, if this should come to trial, would be asked to testify about exactly what the patient said and their perception of whether this was a revoked consent. Good judgment, prudence, and discretion will keep the colonoscopist out of trouble.[21]

STANDARD OF CARE FOR MONITORING SEDATION

If a sedation-related complication occurs, the monitoring done during the procedure will be assessed to determine whether endoscopy personnel were trained, whether monitoring equipment was both appropriate and maintained. Local and State regulations may influence your decisions regarding which personnel should have Advanced Cardiovascular Life Support training. Awareness of changing environment will allow determinations regarding adoption of newer technology, such as decision about using capnography in addition to currently standard blood pressure, pulse oximetry, and cardiac monitoring.[22]

USE OF ANESTHESIA PERSONNEL FOR ENDOSCOPIC SEDATION

Recently, the percentage of colonoscopies and upper endoscopy procedures furnished using an anesthesia professional has increased from 13.5% in 2003 to 30.2% in 2009 within the Medicare population, with a similar increase in the commercially insured population.[23] There are patients whose acuity of illness or physical characteristics are such that they present a high risk for problems during endoscopic procedures. Should an adverse outcome occur, a legal review will involve whether an adequate preprocedure assessment was done (ie, was there a short, thick neck or high American Society of Anesthesiologists classification), and whether the question of an appropriate request to use anesthesia services was made. Some hospital facilities require patients at a certain American Society of Anesthesiologists classification to be sedated with anesthesia. Violating one's own hospital policy is difficult to defend in court. On the other hand, the use of anesthesia personnel does not automatically remove liability risk from the gastroenterologist. In outpatient settings where the gastroenterologist has been involved in selecting the anesthesia personnel to provide care in their ambulatory surgical center, under legal doctrines such as "captain of the ship" and vicarious liability, culpability may attach to the gastroenterologist performing a procedure in which an anesthesiology-related sedation issue arose.[24] However, courts increasingly either reject the "captain of the ship" doctrine in favor of general agency principles over the right to control a negligent actor, or refuse to apply the doctrine in its traditional form.[25]

NEW AGENTS, DEVICES, AND SYSTEMS

Despite a great measure of success, endoscopic sedation remains imperfect. There are patients feeling under-sedated, concerns about adequacy of monitoring systems, and interest in and concern about the widespread adoption of monitored anesthesia care for low-risk patients undergoing routine procedures. This has led to attempts to innovate. Gastroenterologist-directed propofol remains under intense study, with increasing epidemiologic data being collected to assess safety. Those data will have potential legal impact, particularly as protocols are more defined. Computer systems for sedation are also in development, and may influence choice of sedation method if enhanced safety is demonstrated. Recently, the US Food and Drug

Administration approved commercial distribution of a device (SEDASYS) to administer intravenous propofol in adult patients undergoing colonoscopy and esophagogastro-duodenoscopy procedures.[26]

Gastroenterologists will need to evaluate new systems regarding efficacy and risk.

SUMMARY

Gastrointestinal endoscopy has been an important medical advance, and has grown in use and complexity. It remains generally quite safe and well-tolerated, but with some risk. Considerations for risk minimization regarding medicolegal issues have included a review of obtaining informed consent for the sedation as well as the procedure, with special reference to open access endoscopy and the possibility of perceived "under-sedation," and the possible withdrawal of consent during the procedure.

The standard of care for the monitoring of sedation will evolve, and will be used to measure whether sedation was delivered safely if an untoward event occurs. The use of anesthesia personnel to deliver sedation for high-risk patients is widely accepted, and thus is standard of care (although when a patient crosses the line to becoming a high-risk patient may be unclear). The use of anesthesia personnel to deliver sedation for average risk patients remains controversial. New agents, devices and systems will likely be touted to improve not only patient outcomes, but also medicolegal risk.

REFERENCES

1. Aisenberg J, Cohen LB. Sedation in endoscopic practice. Gastrointest Endosc Clin N Am 2006;16:695–708.
2. Lattimore v. Dickey, 239 Cal. App. 4th 959, 968, 191 Cal.Rptr.3d 766, 773 n. 3 (2015).
3. Johnson v. Mid Dakota Clinic, P.C., 864 N.W.2d 269, 273 (N.D. 2015).
4. Swoboda v. Fontanetta, 131 A.D.3d 1042, 1044–45, 17 N.Y.S.3d 50, 53 (2015).
5. See e.g., Laplante v. Rhode Island Hosp., 110 A.3d 261, 265 (R.I. 2015).
6. Nicholson v. Thom, 763 S.E.2d 772, 785–86 (N.C. App. 2014) review denied, 778 S.E.2d 87 (N.C. 2015) (applying res ipsa loquitur to the retained sponge example); See also note 2, supra.
7. See e.g., Halls v. Kiyici, 104 A.D.3d 502, 504–05, 960 N.Y.S.2d 423, 425 (2013) (court should instruct juries that American Gastroenterological Association guide-lines for frequency of colonoscopies are merely treatment recommendations and do not establish standards of care for diagnosis/treatment of colon cancer.).
8. Canterbury v. Spence, 464 F.2d 772, 787–88 (D.C. Cir. 1972); Bradley v. Sugar-baker, — F.3d —, 2015 WL 9095621 (1st Cir. 2015).
9. Aisenberg J, Cohen LB, Piorkowski JD. Propofol use under the direction of trained gastroenterologists: an analysis of the medicolegal implications. Am J Gastroenterol 2007;101:707–13.
10. Cohen L, Delegge M, Aisenberg J, et al. AGA institute review of endoscopic sedation. Gastroenterology 2007;133:675–701.
11. Petrini J, Egan JV. Risk management regarding sedation/analgesia. Gastrointest Endosc Clin N Am 2004;14(2):401–6.
12. Petrini DA, Petrini JD. Risk assessment and management for endoscopists in an ambulatory surgery center. Gastrointest Endosc Clin N Am 2006 Oct;16(4):801–15.
13. Feld AD. Informed consent: not just for procedures anymore. Am J Gastroenterol 2004;99:977–80.
14. Fox v. Kramer, 22 Cal. 4th 531, 994 P.2d 343 (2000).

15. Ward B, Shah S, Kirwan P, et al. Issues of consent in colonoscopy: if a patient says "stop" should we continue? J R Soc Med 1999;92(3):132–3.
16. See Doctors Hosp. of Augusta, LLC v. Alicea, 332 Ga. App. 529, 544–45, 774 S.E.2d 114, 125-26 (2015); Morvillo v. Shenandoah Memorial Hosp., 547 F. Supp. 2d 528, 531 (W.D. Va. 2008).
17. Andrew v. Begley, 203 S.W.3d 165, 172 (Ky. App. 2006) (citing Mims v. Boland, 110 Ga. App. 477, 483-84, 138 S.E.2d 902, 907 (1964)).
18. Bradley v. Sugarbaker, — F.3d —, 2015 WL 9095621 (1st Cir. 2015).
19. Cobbs v. Grant, 8 Cal.3d 229, 240, 502 P.2d 1, 8 (1972).
20. See e.g., Linog v. Yampolsky, 376 S.C. 182, 188, 656 S.E.2d 355, 358 n. 1 (2008) (expressing "serious doubts as to whether a patient could ever revoke consent to a medical procedure while under anesthesia or ... significant sedation.").
21. Feld AD "Informed consent For Colonoscopy" in Waye, Rex, Williams Colonoscopy, in press.
22. Vargo JJ, Ahmad AS, Aslanian HR, et al. Training in patient monitoring and sedation and analgesia. Gastrointest Endosc 2007;66(1):7–10.
23. Liu H, Waxman DA, Main R, et al. Utilization of Anesthesia Services during Outpatient Endoscopies and Colonoscopies and Associated Spending in 2003-2009. JAMA 2012;307(11):1178–84.
24. Cohen, note 10, supra.
25. See Willis v. Bender, 596 F.3d 1244, 1263–64 (10th Cir. 2010) (collecting cases).
26. FDA Notice – Medical Devices; Availability of Safety and Effectiveness Summaries for Premarket Approval Applications; SEDASYS Computer-Assisted Personalized Sedation System (78 Fed. Reg. 50422, August 19, 2013).

Non–Operating Room Anesthesia in the Endoscopy Unit

Sekar Bhavani, MD, MS, FRCS (I)

KEYWORDS

- NORA • NORA patient selection • NORA anesthetic management

KEY POINTS

- The need for non–operating room anesthesia (NORA) increased exponentially in the past decade. This is driven by multiple factors.
- Anesthesiologists are forced to work outside their comfort zone, forcing them to think outside the box.
- Proper preprocedure evaluation and preprocedural optimization of comorbidities as appropriate are key to providing optimal care.

INTRODUCTION

The term, *NORA*, was coined to describe a location remote from the main operating suites and closer to the patient. The American Society of Anesthesiologists (ASA) in its newsletter in November 2013 recognized this transformation in delivery of health care that will continue to push the locus of care closer to the patient and in nontraditional settings.[1] Unlike ambulatory procedures that might be done at designated rooms in the operating room suite, or separate designated building on or off campus,[2] out-of–operating room procedures usually mean procedures carried out in areas that offer specialized procedures, like endoscopy suites, cardiac catheterization laboratories, invasive radiology, and so forth. As both the monitoring technology and anesthetic techniques continue to improve, the number of cases performed at remote locations continue to grow and many institutions have reported that up to 30% of anesthetics are administered to patients outside the operating room.[3]

The need for NORA has increased exponentially in the past decade. This is driven by many factors. Most institutions have areas where the facilities are optimized to provide state-of-the-art diagnostic and therapeutic options for patients. These may involve fixed complex instruments that are impossible to move to an operating suite or might

Institute of Anesthesiology, CCLCM, Cleveland Clinic Main Campus, 9500 Euclid Avenue, Cleveland, OH 44195, USA
E-mail address: bhavans@ccf.org

Gastrointest Endoscopy Clin N Am 26 (2016) 471–483
http://dx.doi.org/10.1016/j.giec.2016.02.007
1052-5157/16/$ – see front matter

involve expensive upgrading of the operating suites to safely facilitate their use. The size or layout of these rooms may not allow for handling the extra equipment required in an already crowded operating room.[4] In some cases, out-of–operating room procedures that are considered minimally invasive are selected as a less risky alternative to an operating room procedure.[5] In other instances, these remote sites may be more efficient and cost saving and provide for better patient and provider satisfaction by bringing together the facility, personnel, and equipment.

The challenges anesthesiologists face are due to an unfamiliar environment and surroundings that result in confusion of the location of equipment and supplies, unavailability of some critical equipment, paucity of space, limited access to the airway due to shared airway or barriers to easy and ready access, increasing complexity of the procedures performed outside the operating room, and increasing patient acuity.[3,6] Anesthesiologists are forced to work and think outside the box, develop new skill sets, and modify anesthetic techniques to provide a safe and smooth anesthetic experience.

There has been such a significant surge in these out-of–operating room procedures that the need for training graduates that addresses these complexities has been recognized by both the American Board of Anesthesiology and the major societies and is being incorporated into the training curriculum at most anesthesia residency programs.[3] But what must be recognized is the need to provide the same levels of safety and standardization that are provided in the operating room environment that have allowed the specialty to succeed. Expansion into this realm should be driven by "what is best" for the patient and not by "what is possible."[7]

SELECTION OF LOCATION

Most of the interventional procedures in the gastrointestinal (GI) suite done before this millennium did not need much anesthesia support; hence, the configuration of the rooms was not designed with the anesthesia provider in mind.[5] In 2009, the Centers for Medicare and Medicaid Services (CMS) Conditions for Coverage eliminated the distinction between a sterile operating room and a nonsterile procedure room. In 2013, the ASA published the standards, guidelines, and policies that should be adhered to in all nonoperating room settings except where they are not applicable to an individual patient or care setting.[8] The goal of these guidelines is to advance NORA to the same level of safety and standardization that is mandated in the operating room environment (**Boxes 1 and 2, Fig. 1**).

Anesthesia outside the operating room is away from the usual operating room environment and, therefore, requires careful monitoring to avoid adverse events. The ASA addressed this issue in their *Statement on Nonoperating Room Anesthetizing Locations*[8] and *Standards for Basic Anesthesia Monitoring*[9] The important guidelines include the following.

SELECTION OF THE ANESTHETIC TECHNIQUE

It is important to recognize that the level of sedation or anesthesia during a procedure is often variable. Some routine diagnostic endoscopic procedures can be performed with minimal or no sedation, but procedures that are more complex are better tolerated when deeper levels of sedation are used. Procedures that are painful or require an absolutely still patient also necessitate a deeper plane of sedation or general anesthesia (GA) with or without instrumentation of the airway.[10]

Nonanesthesiologists sometimes fail to realize that sedation is a continuum and can range from minimal sedation through conscious sedation, deep sedation, and GA.

Box 1

Some important requirements for nonoperating room locations

- Need to observe all applicable building and safety codes and facility standards, where they exist

- Sufficient space to accommodate necessary equipment and personnel and to allow expeditious access to the patient, anesthesia machine (when present) and monitoring equipment

- Sufficient electrical outlets to satisfy anesthesia machine and monitoring equipment requirements, including clearly labeled outlets connected to an emergency power supply

- Isolated electric power or electric circuits with ground fault circuit interrupters in any wet location

- Adequate illumination of the patient, anesthesia machine (when present), and monitoring equipment; battery-powered illumination for backup

Data from ASA. Statement on nonoperating room anesthetizing locations: committee of origin: standards and practice parameters (approved by the ASA house of delegates on October 19, 1994, and last amended on October 16, 2013). ASA; 2013. Accessed 2015.

There is a progressive depression of central nervous system (CNS) with progressive decrease in the levels of consciousness and responsiveness to painful stimuli, loss of protective reflexes, and ultimately depression of the cardiovascular and respiratory system (**Table 1**).[11] There is considerable overlap between the medications used for anxiolysis, conscious and deep sedation, and GA. With adequate doses, a deeper plane of anesthesia may be entered than intended, even when using a medication not designed for deeper planes. In addition, combination of an anxiolytic/sedative and an opioid may produce significant respiratory depression. It is important that when nonanesthesiologists are involved in providing sedation that they should be

---

Box 2

Guidelines from the American Society of Anesthesiologists

- Reliable oxygen source with the piped gases, when available, meeting the applicable codes with a backup supply

- Reliable and adequate source of suction

- An anesthesia machine equivalent in function to that used in operating rooms and maintained to current operating room standards

- Reliable and adequate scavenging of waste anesthetic gases, if applicable

- A self-inflating hand resuscitator

- An adequate supply of anesthesia drugs and equipment for the intended anesthesia care

- Monitoring that adheres to the *Standards for Basic Anesthesia Monitoring*. This includes a pulse oximetry with audible pulse tone and low-threshold alarm, continuous ECG monitoring, automated blood pressure monitoring every 5 minutes or more frequently as indicated, and temperature in cases expected to be associated with significant changes in body temperature. With the use of propofol to provide deep sedation, with or without instrumentation of the airway, the ASA guidelines now recommend the use of end-tidal CO_2 monitoring with an audible alarm for patients undergoing both moderate and deep sedation.

- An emergency cart with a defibrillator, emergency drugs, and other equipment adequate to provide cardiopulmonary resuscitation

---

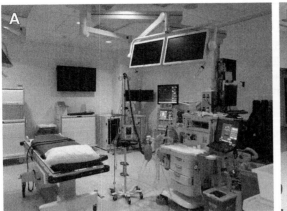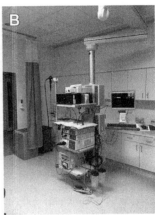

Fig. 1. (*A, B*) Showing the ideal location, space, and orientation for an advanced endoscopy suite.

adequately trained to recognize and rescue patients when they enter a deeper plane of anesthesia than intended.[11]

MEDICATIONS COMMONLY USED FOR ANXIOLYSIS/CONSCIOUS SEDATION

In most institutions in the United States, conscious sedation for endoscopic procedures usually involves the intravenous (IV) bolus administration of a benzodiazepine and a narcotic.[12]

Benzodiazepines

Benzodiazepines stimulate the γ-aminobutyric acid (GABA) receptors (**Table 2**), which results in an increased inhibitory effect of GABA on neuronal excitability.

Table 1
Levels of sedation

	Response	Airway	Cardiovascular System	Neuromuscular Function
Minimal sedation	Normally to verbal commands	Normal	Normal	Normal
Conscious sedation	Purposefully to verbal commands, alone or by light tactile stimulation	Normal	Normal	Normal
Deep sedation	Cannot be easily aroused but responds purposefully after repeated or painful stimulation	May be difficult to maintain	Usually not affected	Normal
GA	Does not respond to painful stimuli	Will need assistance to maintain airway	May be impaired	Depressed

From ASA. Continuum of depth of sedation: definition of general anesthesia and levels of sedation/analgesia*. Committee of origin: quality management and departmental administration (approved by the ASA house of delegates on October 13, 1999, and last amended on October 15, 2014). ASA; 2014.

Table 2
Benzodiazepines

Agent	Route of Administration	Onset of Action	Half-Life	Metabolism
Midazolam GA: 0.1–0.4 mg/kg Sedation 0.01–0.1 mg/kg	Oral/IV/IM/ transnasal	IV—30–60 s IM—15 min Oral—15 min	1–4 h	Liver Metabolites are active but are rapidly cleared.
Diazepam	Oral/IV/IM/ rectal	IV—5 min IM—20–30 min PO—30–60 min	21–37 h	Liver Metabolites are active but slowly cleared.
Lorazepam	Oral/IV/IM	IV—5 min IM—20–30 min PO—30–60 min	10–20 h	Liver Metabolites are inactive.

Abbreviation: IM, intramuscular.

Benzodiazepines produce sedation, anxiolysis, anterograde amnesia, muscle relaxation, and anticonvulsant activity through their effect on the CNS. The commonly used benzodiazepines are midazolam, diazepam, lorazepam, oxazepam, clonazepam, flurazepam, temazepam, triazolam and quazepam, differing in speed of onset and duration of action. They have a ceiling effect that limits CNS depression, but when they are combined with other anesthetic agents, they can lead to profound respiratory depression.

Midazolam is the most commonly selected benzodiazepine for both conscious sedation and as preanesthetic medication. It is a short acting and water-soluble. After an IV bolus, the onset of action is in approximately 30 seconds to 60 seconds, the maximum effect is reached in 3 minutes to 5 minutes, and the effect lasts for 20 minutes to 80 minutes. Termination of action is due to redistribution. It is primarily metabolized in the liver. It duration of action is prolonged with in patients with cirrhosis, congestive heart failure, and renal failure.

Benzodiazepines have dose-dependent cardiorespiratory depressant properties. Midazolam minimally decreases the respiratory rate and tidal volume, but this may become significant if it is given in conjunction with opioids. They should be used with caution in the elderly and in children, in whom it can have a paradoxical effect, and in patients who have hemodynamic instability. Major side effects include confusion, delirium, lightheadedness, motor incoordination, and impairment of cognitive and mental functions.

Flumazenil is a specific benzodiazepine antidote that may antagonize benzodiazepine action. It is a competitive inhibitor of GABA. Duration of antagonism is brief and may require repeated doses. It might, however, trigger seizures, acute withdrawal symptoms, nausea, dizziness, agitation, or arrhythmias in addicts.

Opioids

Opioids comprise a mixed group drugs, both natural and synthetic, that bind to opioid receptors to produce their analgesic effects (**Table 3**). They include the naturally occurring agents, such as morphine, and the synthetic opioids, fentanyl, alfentanil, sufentanil, and remifentanil. Opioids produce a dose-related depression of respiratory

Table 3
Opioids commonly used in the gastrointestinal suite

Opioid	Relative Potency	Time to Onset (min)	Maximum Effect (min)	Half-Life	Metabolism
Meperidine	0.1	2–3	5–7	3–4 h	Liver
Fentanyl	100	2–3	15–20	2–4 h	Liver
Alfentanil	10–25	1.5–2	—	60–90 min	Liver
Sufentanil	500–1000	2	—	2.7 h	Liver
Remifentanil	250	2	1.5–2	5–7 min	Plasma esterases

centers resulting in a decrease in respiratory rate and minute ventilation and an increase in Pco_2.

The receptor specificity determines the effect of the opioids whereas the onset, duration, and effects are determined by the route of administration, absorption, and metabolism.

The factors that increase the sensitivity to opioids include higher doses, concomitant administration of other CNS depressants, anesthetics, respiratory acidosis, decreased hepatic metabolism, and renal failure. Paradoxically, hyperventilation and hypocapnea also increase the effect.

Meperidine

Meperidine is predominantly a μ-opioid receptor agonist with local anesthetic properties. For endoscopic procedures, an initial bolus of meperidine (25 mg) is given and is followed by 25 mg every 3 minutes until the desired level of sedation is achieved. It is metabolized by the liver and excreted by the kidney. The half-life is 3.2 hours to 3.7 hours. The major metabolite normeperidine has analgesic activity and causes muscle twitching and seizures in patients with renal insufficiency due to accumulation. It is contraindicated in patients who are allergic to meperidine and those who are taking monoamine oxidase inhibitors.

Fentanyl

Fentanyl is also is predominantly a μ-opioid receptor agonist. It has a more rapid onset of action and clearance. When given rapidly, it can produce muscular rigidity. It is metabolized by the liver and excreted in the kidneys. When used in conjunction with benzodiazepines, its effect can be potentiated.

MEDICATIONS COMMONLY USED FOR DEEP SEDATION/GENERAL ANESTHESIA
Propofol

Propofol (2,6-diisopropofol) is a sedative-hypnotic drug with an amnestic effect. It has a very short duration of action after an IV bolus. After an induction dose, onset of action occurs in 30 seconds to 60 seconds and duration of effect is 4 minutes to 8 minutes. It is useful in areas where total IV anesthesia is essential when inhaled anesthetic agents cannot be used during sharing the airway or in the absence of a scavenging system. It has minimal analgesic properties. Propofol can cause significant vasodilation and this is more pronounced in the elderly and in patients with reduced intravascular volume. It depresses the breathing and can cause apnea if given rapidly. Propofol is a strong antiemetic, so is ideal in patients who have a history of postoperative and nausea and vomiting. It is important to realize that propofol has a narrow therapeutic range; hence, it is possible to inadvertently enter deeper planes than anticipated. This is complicated by the fact that no reversal for propofol is available. Propofol depresses the respiratory system, so it is required that it be administered only by individuals who are trained in airway management.[13]

There has been controversy regarding the use of propofol by nonanesthesiologists both in the anesthesia and GI literature.[12,14–17] Irrespective of all the controversy that exists, in most institutions anesthesiologists provide oversight and credentialing of sedation practices in the United States.

Dexmedetomidine

Dexmedetomidine is a highly selective α_2-adrenergic agonist. Unlike propofol, it has sedative and analgesic effects. Dexmedetomidine produces a sedation from which the patient can be aroused. It causes minimal respiratory depression. For these reasons, it may be particularly useful in patients with morbid obesity and/or obstructive sleep apnea. Dexmedetomidine can cause bradycardia and hypotension. Usually a loading dose of 1 µg/kg is administered over 10 minutes, followed by an infusion starting at 0.6 µg/kg/h and then titrated to achieve the targeted level of sedation. It has synergistic effects with the other sedatives and opioids, so should be used with caution when combined with other agents.

Ketamine

Ketamine has a rapid onset of action after an IV dose. It produces dissociative anesthesia with significant analgesia properties. It produces minimal respiratory depression and it relaxes bronchial smooth muscle. Ketamine can cause increases in blood pressure, heart rate, and cardiac output by stimulating the sympathetic nervous system centrally. It is, however, a direct cardiac depressant.

Ketamine can produce bad dreams, hallucinations, and out-of-body experiences that cause emergence delirium in adults. This effect can be countered by a preinduction dose of a benzodiazepine. Ketamine increases salivation and this can be problematic in patients undergoing upper GI endoscopy. Premedication with an anticholinergic can limit this effect. It can be used safely in patients who have opioid dependence or addiction.

Ketamine and propofol can been mixed together as ketofol for procedural sedation. When mixed, the dose of ketamine required is greatly reduced, and the risk of postprocedure dysphoria also reduced.

NEWER MEDICATIONS IN THE HORIZON

- Remimazolam is a benzodiazepine derivative now in phase 2 trials. Remimazolam was found to have a faster onset and a shorter duration of action compared with midazolam.
- Fospropofol is a water-soluble prodrug of propofol. It is rapidly hydrolyzed by alkaline phosphatases to propofol. When an equipotent dose is administered, the rise is similar but peak levels are lower and there is an extended plateau phase. After administration of the drug, there is a rapid onset of action and a sustained effect that lasts for 15 minutes to 30 minutes.[18]

ANESTHETIC TECHNIQUES

Patients may undergo GI endoscopic procedures without sedation, analgesia, or both; however, a majority of patients receive some level of sedation and analgesia. Most of the GI procedures can be safely carried out under various levels of sedation without instrumentation of the airway (monitored anesthesia care [MAC]). Failure to recognize the need for securing the airway can result, however, in significant periprocedural mortality and morbidity. One common misconception in the GI community is the association of GA and the presence of an endotracheal tube. Although counterintuitive, the risks of MAC are higher than a GA.[19,20] There are risks associated with intubation or manipulation of the upper airway and they can occur during intubation, during the time when the endotracheal tube is in place, during extubation, or during recovery.

INDICATIONS FOR ANESTHESIA SERVICES

- Emergencies
- Age under 18 years (ie, to the 18th birthday)
- Pregnancy status
- Uncooperative or patients with agitated or altered mental status
- Intolerance to the medications commonly used for moderate sedation (ie, benzodiazepines and/or narcotics)
- Previous problems with sedation or with anesthesia
- History of long-term use/abuse of benzodiazepines, narcotics, alcohol, or neuropsychiatric medications
- Patients with significant cardiac, respiratory (chronic obstructive pulmonary disease), or systemic comorbidities
- ASA class III–IV
- Increased risk for airway obstruction
  - Morbid obesity
  - History sleep apnea
  - Patients with known or suspected difficult airway
  - Airway examination that suggests a difficult intubation
  - Small mouth opening (<3 cm in an adult) or patients after head and neck radiation with a noncompliant submandibular space
  - Micrognathia, retrognathia
- Complex procedures
  - Very long procedure
  - Associated with risk of bleeding
  - Increased risk of regurgitation and aspiration
  - Management of strictures
  - Inflammatory bowel disease
  - Drainage of pseudopancreatic cysts
  - Short bowel syndrome
  - Natural orifice transluminal endoscopic surgeries
- Use of CO_2
- ? Double-balloon upper endoscopies

OTHER ADJUNCTS

- For upper endoscopy, glycopyrrolate can reduce secretions and improve the effectiveness of topical anesthesia. By decreasing the secretions, it may facilitate the local anesthetic action of topical analgesia and also reduce the incidence of laryngospasm.[21]
- Benzocaine spray or topical lidocaine is often used to provide topical anesthesia for upper GI endoscopy cases. A large meta-analysis suggested, "Pharyngeal anesthesia before upper endoscopy improves ease of endoscopy and also improves patient tolerance."[22] Use of topical benzocaine can lead to the development of methemoglobinemia, aspiration, and anaphylactic reactions in susceptible patients.[22]

- Diphenhydramine acts by competing with histamine for H_1-receptor sites, thereby decreasing histamine's actions. It is metabolized in the liver and excreted by the kidneys.
- Droperidol is a neuroleptic agent producing sleep and tranquilization. It was used as premedication and for induction and maintenance of GA. It has antiemetic properties. This drug carries a black box warning from the Food and Drug Administration regarding its use in patients with prolonged T syndrome.

The need for MAC or a GA is to a large extent dictated by the patient age, health status, concurrent medications, preprocedural anxiety, pain tolerance, and procedural variables, such as the degree of invasiveness and the duration of the procedure. The clinician who is ordering the procedure and the one administering the sedation should be familiar with the depth of sedation required for that particular procedure and the patient's comorbidities that might alter the patient's response to sedation and analgesia.

Another advantage for using deep sedation rather than moderate sedation is that patients recover faster because the drug most commonly used to produce deep sedation, propofol, has a better pharmacokinetic and pharmacodynamic profile than the drugs typically used for moderate sedation (midazolam and fentanyl).

PROPER PREPROCEDURE EVALUATION AND PREPROCEDURAL OPTIMIZATION OF COMORBIDITIES

Preprocedural evaluation and preparation are critical to achieve both efficiency and safety in this environment.[5] The ASA has mandated, "The clinicians administering sedation should be familiar with the depth of sedation required for the particular procedure and with aspects of the patient's medical history that might alter the patient's response to sedation and analgesia."[23]

Not uncommonly, the endoscopist providing the services is a consultant and is not the primary provider of care for the patient.[5,21] This leads to paucity of information regarding the comorbidities that need to be considered when triaging these patients to conscious sedation or MAC with the potential to create an adverse outcome. Claims arising from NORA locations have been shown to have a higher proportion of death compared with those from the operating rooms (54% vs 29%, respectively; $P<.001$) and were primarily caused by an adverse respiratory event due to oversedation (44%).[19] GI suites accounted for 32% of these claims. What was more concerning was that they were judged preventable by better monitoring techniques.[19] The JCAHO has mandated guidelines and standards for all institutions to follow. These are virtually identical to requirements for anesthesia care in the operating room. Anesthesiologists have the expertise in perioperative risk stratification of patients and can ensure compliance with standards for presedation assessment. This is an area where the anesthesiologists can step up and provide added value.[24]

The preanesthetic evaluation should at minimum include a review of allergies and current medications, including over-the-counter medications. Prior hospitalizations and surgeries and any adverse outcomes after previous sedation and anesthesia should be elicited and documented. The review of systems should at minimum focus on those conditions that may alter response to the planned sedation. A careful assessment of the airway should be done even in cases that normally would not need airway instrumentation. In addition, a focused examination of the heart, lungs, and neurologic status should be documented. A complete blood cell count and a coagulation profile are warranted in patients with ongoing bleeding or multiple blood transfusions, patients on anticoagulants, or patients with significant liver involvement.

A positive outcome of the preprocedural evaluation is the identification of unresolved medical issues that may need to be addressed prior to the procedure. Involvement or referral to the preanesthesia testing clinic facilitates patient optimization and scheduling and avoids cancellations on the day of the procedure.

PROPER AND APPROPRIATE SELECTION OF THE PROVIDERS
Anesthesia Staff

It is important to realize that not all endoscopies need an anesthesiologist to be included in the care.[25] The anesthesiologist should possess the ability to prevent and treat predictable and unpredictable events. The anesthesiologist should have a working knowledge of the procedure planned. In a majority of instances, because these cases are scheduled on an outpatient basis, the anesthesia provider has to evaluate the patient on the day of the procedure. The development of protocols and guidelines goes a long way to ensure safety and throughputs through a busy endoscopy unit. Patients who require coordination of care between the subspecialties should be evaluated prior to the day of procedure.

Support Staff and Personnel

Education of nonanesthesia personnel in NORA areas is essential. It not only ensures effective throughput through these high-volume rapid turnover locations but also provides safety when emergencies and complication occur because the resources available are often not equivalent to those present in the operating room. Hence, the teams should be focused and efficient and prepared for all possible consequences of NORA.[10]

- Adequate staff trained to support the anesthesiologist.
- Appropriate postanesthesia management should be provided.
- In addition to the anesthesiologist, adequate numbers of trained staff and appropriate equipment should be available to safely transport the patient to a postanesthesia care unit.

Education of Nonanesthesia Personnel for Sedation

It is important that the person involved in sedation should be able to identify, rescue, and manage any complications that might arise due to inadvertent deeper levels of sedation than planned. To this extent, the ASA has developed guidelines for sedation by nonanesthesiology providers.[23,26]

Several other societies, including the American Association for the Study of Liver Diseases, the American College of Gastroenterology, the American Gastroenterological Association, and the American Society for Gastrointestinal Endoscopy, in collaboration with American Association of Nurse Anesthetists, the ASA, and the CMS, have developed sedation curriculum for GI endoscopy.[27]

PROTOCOLS

The continued use of protocols and checklists to enhance safety and define safety standards is an important consideration. The JCAHO has also recognized the need for guidelines and standards for all institutions to follow. These are guidelines and not standard of care. Protocols should facilitate the proper selection of patients by matching location, equipment available, providers, procedure, patient, and the skill sets that the providers bring to the table. These should be a guide that can be used to navigate the clinical challenges encountered but at the same time give the flexibility to respond to the local environment. Implementing protocols across institutions can be a challenge and there is a need for buy-in from the leadership and the authority to negotiate and make decisions. There must be a quality-monitoring system in place to provide feedback, which should be visited often to make changes when it affects patient care.

POSTANESTHESIA CARE

Anesthesiologists have expertise in the perioperative period, so should be actively involved in the management of the airway, oxygenation, ventilation, hemodynamics, pain control, and treatment of nausea in the perioperative period.

Normally, discharge to phase 3 is protocol driven and who should do it should be decided in advance. Protocols for activation of an acute care team in cases of emergencies should also be in place. The arrangements for transfer to a facility capable of handling a patient should be ascertained before the procedure begins, when the procedure is scheduled in a freestanding center. This is also true when the NORA site is remote from the main hospital building. The anesthesiologist should facilitate the stabilization, management, and subsequent admission at least in the initial phase.

Anesthetists in the procedural suite may not have ready access to additional skilled anesthesia personnel should complications occur. A skilled postoperative nursing unit may be required for these complex patients; availability should be ascertained before the procedure begins. In some cases, such a unit may not be available, and planning ahead of time for postprocedure transport to a monitored area or ICU may need to be considered.

COMPLICATIONS OF SEDATION AND ANESTHESIA

Complications of sedation/analgesia are usually due to a deeper plane of anesthesia than anticipated. The loss of airway patency due to airway obstruction or respiratory depression may lead to life-threatening hypoxia and hypercarbia that can result in hypotension and cardiac arrhythmias and depression.[19,20,28,29] In addition, depression of protective airway reflexes due to excessive sedation can lead to an unprotected airway and thereby increases the risk of regurgitation and aspiration of gastric contents.

SUMMARY

Success in the planning and implementation of a NORA involves not only the proper selection of a location to provide the care but also the proper selection of an anesthetic technique, proper preprocedure evaluation, preprocedural optimization of comorbidities as appropriate, and appropriate selection of the provider.

The routine use of anesthesia providers for routine endoscopies is not cost.

Clear communication between GI proceduralist and anesthetist is critical for a good outcome. If it is difficult for proceduralists to anticipate the course of a procedure, it is then impossible for an anesthesia provider to anticipate the course of a procedure when there are procedural difficulties.

REFERENCES

1. Pomerantz P. Report: away from the O.R., and closer to the patient. Newsl Am Soc Anesthesiol 2013;77(11):8–9.
2. Apfelbaum JL, Cutter TW. The four Ps: place, procedure, personnel, and patient. Anesthesiol Clin 2014;32(2):xvii–xxi.
3. Ferrari LR. Anesthesia outside the operating room. Curr Opin Anaesthesiol 2015; 28(4):439–40.

4. Bell C, Sequeira PM. Nonoperating room anesthesia for children. Curr Opin Anaesthesiol 2005;18(3):271–6.
5. Bader AM, Pothier MM. Out-of-operating room procedures: preprocedure assessment. Anesthesiol Clin 2009;27(1):121–6.
6. Dexter F, Wachtel RE. Scheduling for anesthesia at geographic locations remote from the operating room. Curr Opin Anaesthesiol 2014;27(4):426–30.
7. Eichhorn V, Henzler D, Murphy MF. Standardizing care and monitoring for anesthesia or procedural sedation delivered outside the operating room. Curr Opin Anaesthesiol 2010;23(4):494–9.
8. ASA. Statement on nonoperating room anesthetizing locations: committee of origin: standards and practice parameters (approved by the ASA house of delegates on October 19, 1994, and last amended on October 16, 2013). ASA; 2013.
9. ASA. Standards for Basic anesthesia monitoring: committee of origin: standards and practice parameters (approved by the ASA house of delegates on October 21, 1986, last amended on October 20, 2010, and last affirmed on October 28, 2015). ASA; 2015.
10. Michel Foehn ER. Adult and pediatric anesthesia/sedation for gastrointestinal procedures outside of the operating room. Curr Opin Anaesthesiol 2015;28(4):469–77.
11. ASA. Continuum of depth of sedation: definition of general anesthesia and levels of sedation/analgesia* committee of origin: quality management and departmental administration (Approved by the ASA House of Delegates on October 13, 1999, and last amended on October 15, 2014). ASA; 2014.
12. American Association for the Study of Liver Diseases, American College of Gastroenterology, American Gastroenterological Association Institute, et al. Multisociety sedation curriculum for gastrointestinal endoscopy. Gastroenterology 2012;143(1):e18–41.
13. Standards of Practice Committee of the American Society for Gastrointestinal Endoscopy, Lichtenstein DR, Jagannath S, Baron TH, et al. Sedation and anesthesia in GI endoscopy. Gastrointest Endosc 2008;68(5):815–26.
14. Heuss LT, Froehlich F, Beglinger C. Nonanesthesiologist-administered propofol sedation: from the exception to standard practice. Sedation and monitoring trends over 20 years. Endoscopy 2012;44(5):504–11.
15. Guimaraes ES, Campbell EJ, Richter JM. The safety of nurse-administered procedural sedation compared to anesthesia care in a historical cohort of advanced endoscopy patients. Anesth Analg 2014;119(2):349–56.
16. Vargo JJ, Cohen LB, Rex DK, et al. Position statement: nonanesthesiologist administration of propofol for GI endoscopy. Gastrointest Endosc 2009;70(6):1053–9.
17. Vargo JJ, Cohen LB, Rex DK, et al, American Association for the Study of Liver Diseases, American College of Gasteroenterology. Position statement: nonanesthesiologist administration of propofol for GI endoscopy. Gastroenterology 2009;137(6):2161–7.
18. Pambianco DJ. Future directions in endoscopic sedation. Gastrointest Endosc Clin N Am 2008;18(4):789–99, x.
19. Metzner J, Posner KL, Domino KB. The risk and safety of anesthesia at remote locations: the US closed claims analysis. Curr Opin Anaesthesiol 2009;22(4):502–8.
20. Hug CC Jr. MAC should stand for maximum anesthesia caution, not minimal anesthesiology care. Anesthesiology 2006;104(2):221–3.
21. Tetzlaff JE, Vargo JJ, Maurer W. Nonoperating room anesthesia for the gastrointestinal endoscopy suite. Anesthesiol Clin 2014;32(2):387–94.

22. Evans LT, Saberi S, Kim HM, et al. Pharyngeal anesthesia during sedated EGDs: is "the spray" beneficial? A meta-analysis and systematic review. Gastrointest Endosc 2006;63(6):761–6.

23. ASA. Advisory on granting privileges for deep sedation to non-anesthesiologist sedation practitioners- committee of origin: ad hoc on non-anesthesiologist privileging (approved by the ASA house of delegates on October 20, 2010). 2010.

24. Warner ME, Warner MA. The value of sedation by anesthesia teams for complex endoscopy: perhaps not what you'd think. Anesth Analg 2014;119(2):222–3.

25. ASA. Statement on anesthesia care for endoscopic procedures: committee of origin: committee on economics approved by the ASA house of delegates on October 15, 2014. 2014.

26. American Society of Anesthesiologists Task Force on Sedation and Analgesia by Non-Anesthesiologists. Practice guidelines for sedation and analgesia by non-anesthesiologists. Anesthesiology 2002;96(4):1004–17.

27. Vargo JJ, DeLegge MH, Feld AD, et al. Multisociety sedation curriculum for gastrointestinal endoscopy. Am J Gastroenterol 2012. [Epub ahead of print].

28. Robbertze R, Posner KL, Domino KB. Closed claims review of anesthesia for procedures outside the operating room. Curr Opin Anaesthesiol 2006;19(4):436–42.

29. Robinson M, Davidson A. Aspiration under anaesthesia: risk assessment and decision-making. Continuing Education Anaesth Crit Care Pain 2013.

Endoscopist-Directed Propofol

Douglas K. Rex, MD, MACP, MACG, FASGE, AGAF

KEYWORDS

- Propofol • Endoscopist-directed propofol • Nurse administered propofol sedation
- Sedation

KEY POINTS

- Endoscopist-directed propofol (EDP) refers to delivery of propofol for endoscopic sedation under the direction of an endoscopist without any involvement of an anesthesia specialist (anesthesiologist or nurse anesthetist).
- EDP has been proven to be safe and is also cost-effective compared with anesthetist-delivered sedation for endoscopy.
- EDP has been endorsed by US gastroenterology societies as an appropriate paradigm for clinical practice.
- EDP has proliferated in Switzerland and Germany, but its expansion in the United States has been limited by financial disincentives, concerns about medical-legal risk for endoscopists, and regulatory obstacles.

TERMINOLOGY SURROUNDING ENDOSCOPIST-DIRECTED PROPOFOL

Endoscopist-directed propofol (EDP) was a term that developed late in the history of propofol administration without involvement of anesthesia specialists. The term "EDP" was meant in part to emphasize that the process of delivering propofol without the involvement of anesthesia specialists remains under the control of, direction of, and the responsibility of the endoscopist. As such, EDP encompasses and includes the earlier term nurse-administered propofol sedation (NAPS). The introduction of NAPS for endoscopy to the United States is credited to John Walker, a private practice gastroenterologist in Medford, Oregon. With the cooperation and direction of an anesthesiologist working in his surgery center, Dr Walker developed protocols for registered nurses to carefully titrate propofol as a single agent for endoscopic procedures.[1] Many early adopters, including myself, began the administration of propofol without anesthesia specialists by traveling with key nurses to Medford, Oregon, to observe Dr Walker's practice of NAPS.

Conflict of Interest: PAION Medical, research support.
Indiana University Hospital, Room 4100, 550 North University Boulevard, Indianapolis, IN 46202, USA
E-mail address: drex@iu.edu

Gastrointest Endoscopy Clin N Am 26 (2016) 485–492
http://dx.doi.org/10.1016/j.giec.2016.02.010
1052-5157/16/$ – see front matter © 2016 Elsevier Inc. All rights reserved.
giendo.theclinics.com

Despite the remarkable success and safety record of Dr Walker's program, it became clear that propofol as a single agent was very difficult to use outside of deep sedation or general anesthesia. Although some groups have titrated single-agent propofol to moderate sedation, most endoscopists feel that initiating upper endoscopy in a patient sedated with propofol alone while still in moderate sedation results in marked coughing and gagging.[2] The natural impulse is then to administer additional propofol and push the patient into deep sedation or general anesthesia. Colonoscopy with single-agent propofol is safer and easier compared with upper endoscopy,[3] but in moderate sedation with single-agent propofol, colonoscopy patients may posture and move, and the typical inclination is to push the patient into deep sedation. "Balanced propofol sedation" (BPS) was developed specifically to allow propofol to be titrated to moderate sedation.[4] The key to achieving moderate sedation in BPS is to administer a small amount of an opioid and/or benzodiazepine before the first dose of propofol. Some experts have argued that the potential for synergism between drugs in different classes creates excessive risk with combination therapy that should be avoided. However, any such assertion reflects an insufficient experience with using propofol in combination with other agents for procedural sedation, as combination therapy virtually enables the targeting of propofol to moderate sedation.[2,4,5] During upper endoscopy, fentanyl blocks the tendency of patients to cough, and during colonoscopy, fentanyl provides some pain relief, whereas a benzodiazepine (almost always midazolam) provides excellent amnesia for the patient in moderate sedation. Further, the opioid and benzodiazepine block the posturing and withdrawal responses when procedures are performed in moderate sedation with single-agent propofol. During BPS, doses of fentanyl are typically 50 to 75 μg, and midazolam doses are 1 to 2 mg. Following the initial dose of opioid and/or benzodiazepine, all further doses are with propofol. During BPS, both upper endoscopy and colonoscopy can be carried out at the level of the moderate sedation, and the total dose of propofol is usually reduced by half or more compared with the amount of propofol administered as a single agent.[5] Dosing of propofol in BPS is less frequent compared with single-agent propofol, which reduces stress for the individual who is titrating the drug.

In our experience, we settled into a pattern of using BPS for all upper endoscopic procedures and for all colonoscopies that we considered at higher risk for airway obstruction, such as patients with obesity or obstructive sleep apnea. For thin patients with low-risk airways, we often used single-agent propofol for colonoscopy, as the risk of airway obstruction or prolonged apnea in thin patients with low-risk airways during colonoscopy was almost negligible in our experience. This was true despite our consistent targeting of deep sedation when using single-agent propofol. Both NAPS in any format, as well as BPS, are encompassed under the term EDP. The simple requirement for EDP is the administration of propofol by a registered nurse (occasionally by the endoscopist), with supervision by the endoscopist, without any involvement of anesthesia specialists (either an anesthesiologist or a nurse anesthetist).

BASIC PRINCIPLES OF ENDOSCOPIST-DIRECTED PROPOFOL

Whether propofol is used as a single agent or as the core drug in BPS, the basic principles of its administration are similar. In BPS, the doses administered should be approximately half of those used when administering propofol as a single agent. The optimal method of administering propofol to maximize safety in EDP is different from the way I commonly see it used by anesthesiologists. Anesthesia specialists often use propofol as an induction agent in the United States before general anesthesia. As such, they frequently give a single bolus of 100 to 200 mg, which frequently induces coma and apnea. Although I see anesthesia specialists safely administer similar doses when using propofol for endoscopic procedures, this is not the best way to achieve a good safety record in EDP.

The principal factor governing dosing in EDP is that the drug has no reversal agent. If enough propofol is given as a single bolus, one can induce apnea and general anesthesia for a number of minutes, certainly long enough to have a very bad outcome in the absence of effective resuscitation. The key to safety with EDP is to titrate the dose and avoid overshooting as much as possible. If done effectively, cautiously, and with constant monitoring of the sedation level and ventilation, any overshoot will be very brief. In effect, with appropriate caution in the titration of propofol, there is no need for a reversal agent because the short duration of action of propofol ensures a brief duration for any apnea that is induced.

In our practice, we limited initial doses of propofol to 50 mg or less. In small, elderly, or frail patients, and those with multiple comorbidities, initial boluses were commonly 20 to 30 mg. After the initial bolus, a useful rule developed by Ludwig Heuss and colleagues[6] was the 20/20 rule, which is no more than 20 mg of propofol administered at an interval no shorter than every 20 seconds.

Colonoscopy can be done with an initial bolus of propofol followed by an intravenous infusion. However, for upper endoscopy and colonoscopy, our observation was that bolus administration throughout provided the best speed to initial intubation and less likelihood of full arousal during the procedure. As noted, the frequency of bolus administration is reduced and therefore administration is simplified compared with bolus titration with single-agent propofol. Training in procedural sedation is covered elsewhere in this issue (see Ben Da, James Buxbaum: Training and Competency in Sedation Practice, in this issue), but training in EDP should follow recommended training guidelines.[7]

Colonoscopy technique is somewhat different in deep sedation compared with moderate sedation. In particular, there tends to be more reliance on abdominal pressure compared with position change to advance the colonoscope during insertion.[8]

SAFETY HISTORY

In 2010, Rex and colleagues[3] summarized the safety of EDP in 646,080 cases in 28 centers from 10 countries. Previously published experience was cited, but there were also 422,424 previously unpublished patients from these 28 centers. The total number of patients in these prospectively collected series who had required endotracheal intubation was 11, prominent neurologic injuries were recorded in 0, and there were 4 deaths. The 4 patients who died included 2 with pancreatic cancer, a patient with severe cardiomyopathy, and a severely handicapped patient with mental retardation. The overall frequency of patients requiring mask ventilation support during the procedure was 0.1% for patients undergoing upper endoscopy, and 0.01% for colonoscopy, confirming that colonoscopy is a safer procedure for EDP.[3]

In a cost analysis in the article, assuming that anesthesia specialists would have been able to prevent the 4 deaths, the minimum cost per life-year saved for involvement of anesthesia specialists in the cases was estimated to be $5.3 million, confirming that from a safety perspective, the use of anesthesia specialists is not cost-effective.

THE POLITICS OF ENDOSCOPIST-DIRECTED PROPOFOL

Given the strong safety database supporting EDP, it seems natural to ask why the use of EDP did not increase in the United States or even become the main paradigm of procedural sedation. This question suggests that evidence alone drives most or all policies and practices in medicine. Since 2009, the use of EDP in the United States has actually declined, not as a result of medical evidence suggesting that it is unsafe, but primarily because of regulations instituted by the Centers for Medicare and Medicaid Services (CMS).[9] EDP has flourished primarily in Switzerland[3,6,10] and Germany,[11,12] where the financial incentives for an anesthetist's involvement in endoscopy are much lower than in the United States. There still are pockets of EDP in the United States, particularly in hospitals serving socioeconomically disadvantaged populations where again, there is little incentive for an anesthetist's involvement, and in some locations in the US West, where insurers have more effectively restricted the use of monitored anesthesia care (MAC) for routine endoscopic procedures.

The use of MAC, a term that refers to the involvement of an anesthesia specialist to provide procedural sedation regardless of the level of sedation or the agents used to produce sedation, has increased steadily in the United States over the past 15 years,[13] despite the lack of evidence that MAC improves safety. In fact, available evidence indicates that the use of MAC actually *increases* the risk of complications from colonoscopy. In a study in US Medicare patients, there was a statistically significant increased risk of aspiration pneumonia associated with MAC after adjustment for case complexity, and a numerical but not statistically significant increase in perforation risk and splenic injury.[14] In such a study, MAC is a surrogate for propofol use, and the results mean that when patients are deeply sedated or in general anesthesia for colonoscopy, they lose their protective reflexes, and some of them will aspirate. Most of these patients develop only fever or cough and can be treated expectantly or with antibiotics with or without hospitalization.[15] Life-threatening aspiration associated with propofol use is extremely rare. Currently, there is no population-based study that has identified any actual benefit for MAC with regard to a "hard" outcome. This includes no evidence that MAC improves detection of polyps,[16–20] or that it decreases complications. With regard to aspiration, the increased risk is certainly not the result of using an anesthetist, but the consequences of propofol itself. This increased risk of aspiration with propofol and deep sedation cannot apparently be overcome by having an airway specialist present in a patient who has lost airway protective reflexes and is not intubated.

Given the lack of evidence that MAC improves outcomes, and given its substantial costs, why does MAC use in the United States continue to rise? The main drivers for the increasing use of propofol, and specifically its administration by MAC, are patient satisfaction and financial gain. Considerable evidence indicates that many patients find the propofol experience superior to that of opioids and benzodiazepines.[21,22] This is not all patients, because many have a very satisfactory experience with moderate sedation using opioids and benzodiazepines, and a small minority actually prefers unsedated colonoscopy. Nevertheless, many colonoscopists use propofol delivered by MAC for essentially all procedures. The main driver with regard to patient satisfaction is the continuous and ongoing observation of delighted patients in the recovery area who felt no pain, are wide awake, and are not nauseated. In contrast, some patients receiving opioids and benzodiazepines experience discomfort (though they seldom remember it), some feel poorly after the procedure, including nausea and vomiting in a few, and some feel that they have lost an entire day or more to the after effects of opioid and benzodiazepine sedation. Given this constant reinforcement of high patient satisfaction with propofol, many endoscopists conclude that everyone will be happier if they receive propofol for sedation. Thus, even centers in which the endoscopist has no potential for financial gain associated with MAC (eg, academic centers and centers where endoscopists are employees of hospital systems) often settle on the use of MAC for all or nearly all patients.

In addition to improved satisfaction, the use of MAC provides the opportunity for a very substantial income stream to many endoscopists.[9] The usual strategy is to employ the anesthesia specialist on a salary, or to pay him or her a set fee per procedure, and the endoscopist takes over the billing for the anesthesia services. The difference in the amount billed and the amount paid to the anesthetist becomes an income stream for the endoscopist that can rival or even exceed the professional fees collected from performance of the endoscopy. This approach is considered repugnant to some, but it is legal and is used in many business models. The combination of patient satisfaction and substantial income combine to outweigh the downsides of no improvement in safety and the overall increasing cost to the health care system from the expansion of MAC.

Why MAC instead of EDP? First, there is no financial incentive for any party in EDP, because the cost of administering sedation for endoscopic procedures is considered part of the standard professional fee, as it is for bronchoscopy and many cardiac procedures. In addition, many endoscopists perceive EDP as a very significant medical-legal risk. This is based first on the package insert statement that propofol should be administered only by persons trained in general anesthesia. The propofol package insert was created entirely before the publication of excellent safety with EDP, but endoscopists reckon that the package insert would still enter into a medical-legal action against an endoscopist practicing EDP. Next is the position of the American Society of Anesthesiology (ASA), which states that deep sedation is the purview of anesthesia specialists only, and that propofol by definition is an agent for deep sedation.[23] Although the ASA has obvious financial conflicts of interest with regard to their sedation policies, and has a history of creating non–evidenced-based position statements that glaringly reflect those conflicts,[9] and despite the evidence that propofol can be titrated to moderate sedation in a balanced propofol regimen,[2] many endoscopists feel certain that plaintiffs' attorneys will have no trouble identifying an anesthesiologist to testify against them in an EDP-related event.

To add to these deterrents to EDP, in December 2009 the CMS issued an "interpretive guideline" stating that only a trained medical doctor or osteopath not involved in the performance of a procedure could administer deep sedation or general anesthesia for procedural sedation, essentially echoing a 2006 ASA House of Delegates statement regarding deep sedation.[9] There is some evidence that CMS was lobbied to create the guideline by the American Association of Nurse Anesthetists[9] and virtually no evidence that CMS either reviewed the literature on EDP, or consulted either emergency room physicians, endoscopists, or other physicians with experience supervising propofol administration without involvement of anesthesia specialists. There was no public comment period before the December 2009 CMS decree (none is required for an "interpretive guideline"). The backlash was considerable, including from emergency department physicians, who effectively established that they are fully trained in airway management. In January 2011, CMS issued a new guideline exempting emergency department physicians from the restrictions. They also stated that other groups of physicians including endoscopists could use any agent (propofol was no longer specifically excluded) in a manner complying with their own national society guidelines,[24] although the 2011 version continued to state that deep sedation is the purview of anesthetists.[9] This revision would appear to allow endoscopists to administer EDP again, provided that they could produce institutional policies consistent with the national guidelines[24] (essentially using BPS targeted to moderate sedation), and provided they could overcome the ongoing ASA policy that propofol equates to deep sedation. Certainly this ASA policy could interfere with the creation of institutional policies. In our own instance, hospital lawyers became a significant deterrent, as the 2009

CMS interpretive guideline is effectively a regulation, and hospitals must comply with all CMS regulations to avoid jeopardizing reimbursement for treating Medicare patients.

I am aware of some hospitals that have created policies that allow EDP, but the obstacles remain substantial. Bizarrely, the CMS regulation was issued for hospitals and never subsequently issued for ambulatory surgery centers and office practices, even though it is obvious that there are fewer airway specialists who can respond to an oversedation situation in those settings compared with hospitals.

In summary, EDP is on the wrong side of financial incentives, is still viewed by endoscopists as a medical-legal risk, and is opposed by the ASA and often by anesthesiologists and nurse anesthetists at the institutional level.

THE FUTURE

The evidence base to support the safety of EDP remains strong, and EDP provides the opportunity to achieve the patient satisfaction benefits of propofol at enormously lower costs than MAC. There is no question that persons involved in administration of EDP need proper training. EDP continues to be an important model for endoscopic sedation in countries in which the obstacles such as those noted previously in the United States are not present. For things to change in the United States, it is likely that MAC would need to become an economic burden to endoscopists, rather than its current status as an economic advantage or being financially neutral. New models for endoscopy reimbursement, such as bundled payment[25] and reference payment[26] that have been proposed and implemented for colonoscopy, have the potential to change the financial incentives around MAC and EDP. However, the MAC lobby, which includes both the anesthesia community and the many endoscopists who profit from MAC, are a powerful force. Time will tell whether medical evidence and payment models that emphasize accountability can overcome this MAC lobby. In the interim, the safety experience with EDP will continue to accumulate in countries in which the EDP model is politically and economically more feasible.

SUMMARY

A substantial evidence base supports the safety of EDP. EDP is cost-effective compared with administration of propofol by anesthesia specialists. Although EDP has successfully expanded in some European countries, its use in the United States has been limited by lack of financial disincentives, concerns about medical-legal risk, and nonevidence based policies of the ASA and CMS.

REFERENCES

1. Walker JA, McIntyre RD, Schleinitz PF, et al. Nurse-administered propofol sedation without anesthesia specialists in 9152 endoscopic cases in an ambulatory surgery center. Am J Gastroenterol 2003;98:1744–50.
2. Rex DK. Review article: moderate sedation for endoscopy: sedation regimens for non- anaesthesiologists. Aliment Pharmacol Ther 2006;24:163–71.
3. Rex DK, Deenadayalu VP, Eid E, et al. Endoscopist-directed administration of propofol: a worldwide safety experience. Gastroenterology 2009;137:1229–37 [quiz: 518–9].
4. Cohen LB, Dubovsky AN, Aisenberg J, et al. Propofol for endoscopic sedation: a protocol for safe and effective administration by the gastroenterologist. Gastrointest Endosc 2003;58:725–32.

5. VanNatta ME, Rex DK. Propofol alone titrated to deep sedation versus propofol in combination with opioids and/or benzodiazepines and titrated to moderate sedation for colonoscopy. Am J Gastroenterol 2006;101:2209–17.
6. Heuss LT, Drewe J, Schnieper P, et al. Patient-controlled versus nurse-administered sedation with propofol during colonoscopy. A prospective randomized trial. Am J Gastroenterol 2004;99:511–8.
7. Vargo JJ, DeLegge MH, Feld AD, et al. Multisociety sedation curriculum for gastrointestinal endoscopy. Gastrointest Endosc 2012;76:e1–25.
8. Hansen JJ, Ulmer BJ, Rex DK. Technical performance of colonoscopy in patients sedated with nurse-administered propofol. Am J Gastroenterol 2004;99:52–6.
9. Rex DK. Effect of the Centers for Medicare & Medicaid Services policy about deep sedation on use of propofol. Ann Intern Med 2011;154:622–6.
10. Heuss LT, Schnieper P, Drewe J, et al. Risk stratification and safe administration of propofol by registered nurses supervised by the gastroenterologist: a prospective observational study of more than 2000 cases. Gastrointest Endosc 2003; 57:664–71.
11. Riphaus A, Stergiou N, Wehrmann T. Sedation with propofol for routine ERCP in high-risk octogenarians: a randomized, controlled study. Am J Gastroenterol 2005;100:1957–63.
12. Wehrmann T, Grotkamp J, Stergiou N, et al. Electroencephalogram monitoring facilitates sedation with propofol for routine ERCP: a randomized, controlled trial. Gastrointest Endosc 2002;56:817–24.
13. Inadomi JM, Gunnarsson CL, Rizzo JA, et al. Projected increased growth rate of anesthesia professional-delivered sedation for colonoscopy and EGD in the United States: 2009 to 2015. Gastrointest Endosc 2010;72:580–6.
14. Cooper G, Kou TD, Rex DK. Complications following colonoscopy with anesthesia assistance: a population-based analysis. JAMA Intern Med 2013;173: 551–6.
15. Friedrich K, Scholl SG, Beck S, et al. Respiratory complications in outpatient endoscopy with endoscopist-directed sedation. J Gastrointestin Liver Dis 2014; 23:255–9.
16. Bannert C, Reinhart K, Dunkler D, et al. Sedation in screening colonoscopy: impact on quality indicators and complications. Am J Gastroenterol 2012;107: 1837–48.
17. Radaelli F, Meucci G, Sgroi G, et al. Technical performance of colonoscopy: the key role of sedation/analgesia and other quality indicators. Am J Gastroenterol 2008;103:1122–30.
18. Paspatis GA, Tribonias G, Manolaraki MM, et al. Deep sedation compared with moderate sedation in polyp detection during colonoscopy: a randomized controlled trial. Colorectal Dis 2011;13:e137–44.
19. Metwally M, Agresti N, Hale WB, et al. Conscious or unconscious: the impact of sedation choice on colon adenoma detection. World J Gastroenterol 2011;17: 3912–5.
20. Wang A, Hoda KM, Holub JL, et al. Does level of sedation impact detection of advanced neoplasia? Dig Dis Sci 2010;55:2337–43.
21. Sipe BW, Rex DK, Latinovich D, et al. Propofol versus midazolam/meperidine for outpatient colonoscopy: administration by nurses supervised by endoscopists. Gastrointest Endosc 2002;55:815–25.
22. Ulmer BJ, Hansen JJ, Overley CA, et al. Propofol versus midazolam/fentanyl for outpatient colonoscopy: administration by nurses supervised by endoscopists. Clin Gastroenterol Hepatol 2003;1:425–32.

23. Policies and Procedures Governing Anesthesia Privileging in Hospitals. Available at: http://www.asahq.org/search?q=Statement%20on%20granting%20privileges %20to%20non-anesthesiologist%20practitioners%20for%20personally%20 administering%20deep%20sedation%20or%20supervising%20deep%20sedation %20by%20individuals%20who%20are%20not%20anesthesia%20professionals. Accessed April 05, 2016.

24. Vargo JJ, Cohen LB, Rex DK, et al. Position statement: nonanesthesiologist administration of propofol for GI endoscopy. Gastrointest Endosc 2009;70: 1053–9.

25. Brill JV, Jain R, Margolis PS, et al. A bundled payment framework for colonoscopy performed for colorectal cancer screening or surveillance. Gastroenterology 2014;146:849–53.e9.

26. Robinson JC, Brown TT, Whaley C, et al. Association of reference payment for colonoscopy with consumer choices, insurer spending, and procedural complications. JAMA Intern Med 2015;175:1783–9.

Extended Monitoring during Endoscopy

Nadim Mahmud, MD, MS, MPH[a], Tyler M. Berzin, MD, MS[b],*

KEYWORDS

- Gastrointestinal endoscopic sedation • Monitoring • Ventilation • Oxygenation
- Hemodynamics • Continuous electrocardiography • Pulse oximetry • Capnography
- Bispectral index

KEY POINTS

- Endoscopic sedation improves procedure outcomes but carries a risk of adverse cardio-pulmonary outcomes.
- Extended monitoring is designed to reduce sedation-associated adverse events through visual assessment and monitors of physiologic parameters.
- Although the evidence base is limited, the American Society of Anesthesiologists and the American Society of Gastrointestinal Endoscopy recommend direct visual assessment, heart rate and blood pressure monitoring, pulse oximetry, and capnography during endoscopic sedation.
- High-risk patients and those requiring deep sedation warrant more intensive monitoring.
- Several novel techniques are emerging and undergoing study to improve monitoring of ventilation and depth of sedation.

BACKGROUND

Endoscopic sedation improves technical procedure quality while reducing patient discomfort[1] and is now used nearly universally for gastroenterologic endoscopic procedures in the United States.[2] Depending on the agent and dose administered, 4 levels of sedation may be achieved: minimal sedation (anxiolysis), moderate sedation (ie, conscious sedation), deep sedation, and general anesthesia. According to the American Society of Anesthesiologists (ASA), these stages should be viewed as a fluid continuum[3,4] and are defined by patients' degree of spontaneous ventilation, maintenance of cardiovascular function, and response to verbal and tactile stimuli (**Table 1**).

Disclosure Statement: This article was jointly written and edited by T. Berzin and N. Mahmud. The authors do not have any funding sources or conflicts of interest to disclose.
[a] Department of Internal Medicine, Brigham and Women's Hospital, Harvard Medical School, 75 Francis Street, Boston, MA 02115, USA; [b] Center for Advanced Endoscopy, Beth Israel Deaconess Medical Center, Harvard Medical School, 330 Brookline Avenue, Boston, MA, USA
* Corresponding author.
E-mail address: tberzin@bidmc.harvard.edu

Gastrointest Endoscopy Clin N Am 26 (2016) 493–505
http://dx.doi.org/10.1016/j.giec.2016.02.006
1052-5157/16/$ – see front matter © 2016 Elsevier Inc. All rights reserved.

Table 1 The sedation continuum				
	Minimal Sedation	**Moderate Sedation**	**Deep Sedation**	**General Anesthesia**
Responsiveness	Normal response to verbal stimulation	Purposeful response to verbal or tactile stimulation	Purposeful response following repeated or painful stimulation	Not able to be aroused even with painful stimulus
Airway	Unaffected	No intervention required	Intervention may be required	Intervention often required
Spontaneous ventilation	Unaffected	Adequate	May be inadequate	Frequently inadequate
Cardiovascular function	Unaffected	Usually maintained	Usually maintained	May be impaired

Adapted from American Society of Anesthesiologists. Continuum of depth of sedation: definition of general anesthesia and levels of sedation/analgesia. 2009. Available at: http://www.asahq.org/~/media/Sites/ASAHQ/Files/Public/Resources/standards-guidelines/continuum-of-depth-of-sedation-definition-of-general-anesthesia-and-levels-of-sedation-analgesia.pdf. Accessed December 23, 2015.

The concept of sedation as a continuum is crucial, as patients may easily and inadvertently drift beyond intended sedation targets and require rescue to restore ventilatory or cardiovascular function.

Sedating and analgesic medications are not without hazard. Opiates, benzodiazepines, and propofol alter one's level of consciousness, depress spontaneous ventilation, and increase cardiopulmonary risk. In a retrospective analysis involving 324,737 patients undergoing endoscopic sedation, Sharma and colleagues[5] found that 0.9% of cases overall were associated with an unplanned cardiopulmonary complication, with higher incidence in more complicated procedures (esophagogastroduodenoscopy [EGD] 0.6%, colonoscopy 1.1%, endoscopic retrograde cholangiopancreatography [ERCP] 2.1%). Risk factors for these adverse events included ASA class III or greater (**Table 2**), advanced age, inpatient status, and trainee involvement in the procedure.

Recognizing the importance of preventing sedation-associated complications, there is great interest in determining the best practices for extended monitoring during endoscopy. In principle, the goal should be to titrate sedatives or anesthetics to the

Table 2 American Society of Anesthesiologists' physical status classification system	
ASA I	Normal healthy patients
ASA II	Patients with mild systemic disease
ASA III	Patients with severe systemic disease
ASA IV	Patients with severe systemic disease that is a constant threat to life
ASA V	Moribund patients who are not expected to survive without the operation
ASA VI	Declared brain-dead patients whose organs are being removed for donor purposes

Adapted from American Society of Anesthesiologists. ASA physical status classification system. 2014. Available at: http://www.asahq.org/resources/clinical-information/asa-physical-status-classification-system. Accessed December 23, 2015.

minimal amount necessary to achieve patient comfort and safety for the endoscopic procedure. As individuals vary in their response to sedating medications, vigilant monitoring is, therefore, required. The major components for effective sedation monitoring include both *appropriate personnel* and *monitors of physiologic parameters*, including hemodynamics, oxygenation, ventilation, and depth of sedation. In the present article, the authors review the evidence base for extended monitoring practices as well as key guidelines and recommendations from the American Society for Gastrointestinal Endoscopy (ASGE) and the ASA (**Table 3**).

DIRECT MONITORING AND PERSONNEL

All patients undergoing sedation during endoscopy must be directly monitored by a trained member of the endoscopy team for the duration of the procedure. *Direct monitoring* refers to both visual assessment of patients as well as review of hemodynamic data collected in real-time through medical devices. Visual assessment may include observing respiratory patterns, depth of chest rise, skin and mucosal coloration, level of consciousness, and facial expressions as a reflection of patient stability and comfort. Devices that monitor relevant hemodynamic parameters are discussed in detail later. In all cases, direct monitoring should begin immediately before the administration of sedation and should continue through procedural recovery. Patients who require agents such as naloxone or flumazenil for opiate or benzodiazepine reversal, respectively, may require several hours of subsequent observation.[6]

The personnel requirements for direct monitoring during endoscopic sedation depend on the depth of sedation and procedural complexity. Although the Joint Commission does not define specific degree qualifications or levels of education for a direct monitoring assistant,[7] the ASGE recommends a registered nurse (RN) with appropriate training for patients receiving moderate sedation.[8] This training should include a working knowledge of the stages of sedation, the skills to monitor and interpret physiologic parameters related to sedation, and the ability to initiate appropriate interventions in the event of a complication.[9] The assistant must be certified in basic or advanced cardiac life support (ACLS). According to a 2006 nationwide survey, RNs are responsible for direct monitoring in approximately 90% of endoscopy sites in the United States.[2]

Table 3
Summary of recommendations from the American Society of Anesthesiologists and American Society for Gastrointestinal Endoscopy for endoscopic monitoring

	ASA[4,13,36]	ASGE[9,12]
Year Updated	2015	2014
Heart rate and blood pressure measurement	Required	Required
Continuous electrocardiography	Required	Required
Pulse oximetry	Required	Required
Capnography	Required for both moderate and deep sedation unless precluded or invalidated by the nature of the patient, procedure, or equipment	Insufficient evidence to recommend for moderate sedation, may consider for deep sedation
Assessment of sedation depth	Required	Required

During moderate sedation cases, a single assistant (typically an RN) may perform direct patient monitoring as well as brief assistive tasks for the endoscopist, such as endoscopic biopsy or application of abdominal pressure. Complex endoscopic cases, such as ERCP or endoscopic ultrasound (EUS)/fine-needle aspiration, should include an additional team member whose sole purpose is technical assistance in order to allow the RN to exclusively focus on direct patient monitoring and administration of sedation. The additional technical member may be an RN, licensed practical nurse (LPN), or unlicensed assistive person (UAP) who has received appropriate training. In these cases there should be at least one additional ACLS certified member of the team who has the ability to secure an airway and provide bag mask ventilation if needed (this is generally the endoscopist).[10] Finally, in cases that include an anesthesia provider, either an anesthesiologist or a certified registered nurse anesthetist, that individual will assume complete responsibility for direct monitoring and an RN, LPN, or UAP may be enlisted to provide technical endoscopic assistance if indicated.

HEMODYNAMIC MONITORING
Heart Rate and Blood Pressure Monitoring

Routine measurement of heart rate and blood pressure is critically important to assess patients' cardiovascular stability before, during, and after an endoscopic procedure requiring intravenous sedation. For example, tachycardia before the case might indicate anxiety, pain, or hypovolemia, especially in patients with significant dehydration after a colonoscopy prep. If a patient becomes hypotensive during the procedure, this could signify excessive sedation (particularly if associated with bradycardia) or hypovolemia. Conversely, intraprocedural hypertension or tachycardia are frequently manifestations of pain or discomfort and suggest insufficient sedation. Changes in these hemodynamic cues allow for early recognition of developing instability and may prompt interventions, such as intravenous fluid boluses, adjustment of sedating medications, or initiation of vasopressor agents.

To date there is only one randomized control trial that addressed the impact of noninvasive hemodynamic monitoring in gastrointestinal endoscopy. DiSario and colleagues[11] randomized 681 individuals undergoing upper endoscopy or colonoscopy to either heart rate and blood pressure monitoring or visual assessment alone. Hemodynamic aberrations were noted in 71% of monitored patients, but there was no difference in adverse events between the groups. Although there is no definitive literature to support the use of heart rate and blood pressure monitoring, this practice is required by both the ASA[4] and the ASGE for cases targeting at least moderate sedation and is considered to be the standard of care.[12] Both organizations recommend automated noninvasive blood pressure cuffs to determine the systolic, diastolic, and mean arterial pressure. Cuff pressures should be cycled every 3 to 5 minutes, with audible tones used if available to indicate if the values have deviated from predefined acceptable ranges.

Electrocardiography

The intended role of continuous electrocardiography during sedation was to detect arrhythmias in patients undergoing deep or general anesthesia. The ASA recommends that continuous electrocardiography be used in any patient receiving sedation.[13] The ASGE shares this recommendation, especially in patients receiving moderate sedation who are elderly, have significant pulmonary disease, or who are undergoing a protracted procedure.[9] Although these recommendations reflect standard practice, no controlled trials to date have addressed the efficacy of cardiac monitoring in endoscopic sedation.[14]

MONITORING OXYGENATION
Pulse Oximetry

Pulse oximetry is a noninvasive means of estimating the oxygen saturation of arterial blood (SaO_2). Modern pulse oximeters consist of a probe with 2 photodiodes and a photodetector. Light is emitted from the photodiodes at 660 nm and 940 nm, wavelengths that correspond to absorption profiles of deoxygenated and oxygenated hemoglobin, respectively.[15] By detecting the relative penetration of these wavelengths at the photodetector while adjusting for pulsatility, the SaO_2 can be calculated.

There are several pitfalls and caveats to note with pulse oximetry. First, at the upper limit of the oxyhemoglobin dissociation curve, large changes in partial pressure of oxygen will only result in small changes in SaO_2. This point is especially true in patients receiving supplemental oxygen, as this shifts the oxyhemoglobin dissociation curve to the left.[16] Second, SaO_2 readings from pulse oximetry are delayed surrogates for hypoxemia, in some cases by more than 50 seconds.[17] This factor is influenced by probe placement,[17] cardiac output, peripheral vasoconstriction, and metabolic factors.[18]

Although no studies have evaluated the impact of pulse oximeter monitoring in patients undergoing endoscopic sedation, several have addressed this in the perioperative setting. The largest was a Danish study by Moller and colleagues[19] who randomized 20,802 patients to pulse oximetry or not. There was a 19-fold increase in the incidence of diagnosed hypoxemia in the intervention arm ($P<.00001$), but no difference in postoperative complications was observed. A 2014 Cochrane review of 5 studies showed increased detection of hypoxemia as well as intraoperative adjustments to patient care. There was no difference in morbidity or mortality.[20]

Despite the limited evidence base in the literature, the ASGE recommends that pulse oximetry be used in any patient for whom the target is at least moderate sedation.[12] The ASA Task Force notes that hypoxemia is more likely to be detected by pulse oximetry than visual assessment alone and recommends that it be used for any patient receiving sedation/analgesia.[4] If available, monitors with variable pitch alarms should be used to increase the recognition of concerning changes in oxygenation. These practice recommendations have become the standard in most endoscopy centers throughout the world, as it is presumed that the data acquired through pulse oximetry ultimately reduce the rate of sedation-associated complications.[21]

MONITORING VENTILATION
Pulse Oximetry

Although the primary purpose of pulse oximetry is to detect hypoxemia, during procedural sedation it is often used as a proxy for ventilation. It is important to recognize that SaO_2 is an indirect and highly insensitive marker of alveolar ventilation, as SaO_2 only decreases once alveolar and arterial carbon dioxide (CO_2) ($PaCO_2$) levels have increased significantly. Further confounding the picture, supplemental oxygen will preserve SaO_2 even in the face of markedly abnormal ventilation.[22] As discussed in greater detail later, pulse oximetry is inferior in detecting hypoventilation as compared with alternative techniques, such as capnography.

Capnography

Capnography is a continuous, noninvasive, real-time means of measuring exhaled CO_2 as a proxy for arterial CO_2 levels ($PaCO_2$). Unlike pulse oximetry, capnography is a direct marker of alveolar ventilation, as exhaled CO_2 levels increase when respiratory status is depressed. Modern capnographs operate on the principle that CO_2 absorbs wavelengths of light in the infrared spectrum. A 4260-nm beam is directed through a sample of exhaled gas, and a sensor detects the intensity of light that remains.[23] These data are used to graph exhaled CO_2 as a function of time, which can be used to detect breath-to-breath variation in ventilation as well as identify abnormal respiratory patterns. Capnographs are available in 2 varieties: mainstream and sidestream. Mainstream devices are used in intubated patients and are inserted between the endotracheal tube and breathing circuit, sampling CO_2 directly in the airway. Sidestream devices can be used in nonintubated patients and function by continuously aspirating gas through either nasal cannula tubing or a dedicated port placed in the mouth. In this case, the CO_2 sampling and analysis occur in the monitor itself rather than the airway.[24]

Studies have demonstrated that capnography offers an earlier indication of hypoventilation as compared with pulse oximetry[25] and is better than visual assessment alone.[26] In the monitored anesthesia setting, it is also efficient in detecting apneic events. Capnography was first used to track ventilation of intubated patients under general anesthesia. Its use has since expanded to monitoring during moderate and deep sedation, including gastrointestinal endoscopic sedation.[27]

The role of capnography in endoscopic sedation has been actively studied in recent years. Cacho and colleagues[28] used both capnography and pulse oximetry in 50 patients undergoing colonoscopy and documented apneas, hypoventilation, and hypoxemic events. Capnography was found to be more reliable in the detection of alveolar hypoventilation, with a mean delay of 38.6 seconds in the detection of hypoventilation through hypoxemia. A meta-analysis of 5 studies using procedural sedation found that capnography led to a 17.6-fold increased likelihood of detecting respiratory depression.[29] Qadeer and colleagues[30] found that capnography usage in complicated endoscopic procedures (ERCP and EUS) led to a lower percentage of hypoxemic events (46% vs 69%, $P<.001$), severe hypoxemia (15% vs 31%, $P = .004$), and apneas (41% vs 63%, $P<.001$). These findings have been replicated in patients undergoing colonoscopy with propofol sedation[31] and in a range of pediatric endoscopic procedures.[32] Despite the improved detection of hypoventilation and prevention of hypoxemia, there remains no evidence that routine capnography improves morbidity or mortality. Koniaris and colleagues[33] retrospectively reviewed 4846 endoscopic procedures using moderate sedation and found that capnography did not significantly modify anesthesia-related complications or morbidity ($P = .3$).

Taken together, the data suggest that capnography may reduce intraprocedural risk in complex cases or in those requiring deeper sedation. In a 2009 joint position statement from the American Association for the Study of Liver Diseases, American Gastroenterological Association, American College of Gastroenterology, and the ASGE, capnography is recommended in prolonged cases, such as EUS/ERCP, or in cases whereby visual assessment is difficult.[34] The same group noted in 2012 that routine capnography in moderate sedation does not improve safety or clinical outcomes but does significantly increase health care costs.[35] Consistent with the aforementioned data, the latest guidelines from the ASGE state that capnography may be considered for cases targeting deep sedation; but there is insufficient evidence to recommend routine capnography in moderate sedation endoscopy.[12] The ASA maintained a similar position until 2011, when an amended statement was released to mandate end-tidal CO_2 monitoring in both moderate and deep sedation procedures.[36] In all cases, societies emphasize that oxygenation and ventilation are separate processes and monitoring one is not a substitute for the other.

MONITORING DEPTH OF SEDATION
Direct Clinical Assessment

Administration of sedating medications may achieve various levels of depressed consciousness. Besides the ASA's continuum of sedation mentioned previously, there are several sedation scales and scoring systems that are used in both the clinical and research setting. The Modified Observer's Assessment of Alertness/Sedation (MOAA/S) Scale is a 5-point scale (5 = fully alert, 0 = no response to pain) that is based on responsiveness to voice and touch, speech, facial expression, and eye ptosis.[37] The Modified Ramsay Sedation Scale (RSS) is an 8-point scale informed by degree of responsiveness to verbal and tactile stimulus (1 = awake and alert, 8 = unresponsive to painful stimulus).[38] These scales are summarized in **Table 4**. To date there have been no studies directly comparing the validity of one sedation scale with another. Both the ASA and ASGE recommend that a trained individual separate from the endoscopist regularly monitor the level of consciousness and sedation stage of patients,[4,12] although there is no specified methodology for this assessment.

Bispectral Index Monitoring

Bispectral (BIS) index monitoring is a noninvasive, objective method of determining level of consciousness using a series of continuous electroencephalogram (EEG) parameters. The monitor uses an algorithm to generate a single index value from 0 (coma) to 100 (fully awake).[39] A BIS index of 80 to 85 is thought to be a reasonable target for moderate sedation in many endoscopy cases.[40] Its potential utility lies in the fact that clinical assessment of depth of sedation—as determined through various scoring systems, such as the MOAA/S or RSS—may be inadequate.

Improved detection and control over sedation targets might theoretically minimize sedative dosing, hemodynamic complications, and shorten patient recovery time.

Table 4	
Formal sedation scales used in clinical and research practice	
MOAA/S	**RSS**
5: Responds readily to name spoken in normal tone	1: Awake and alert, minimal or no cognitive impairment
4: Lethargic response to name spoken in normal tone	2: Awake but tranquil, purposeful responses to verbal commands at a conversational level
—	3: Appears asleep, purposeful response to verbal commands at a conversational level
3: Responds after name called loudly or repeatedly or both	4: Appears asleep, purposeful responses to commands but at a louder than conversational level, requiring light glabellar tap, or both
2: Responds only after mild prodding or mild shaking	5: Asleep, sluggish purposeful responses only to loud verbal commands, strong glabellar tap, or both
1: Responds only to painful stimulation	6: Asleep, sluggish purposeful responses only to painful stimuli
—	7: Asleep, reflex withdrawal to painful stimuli only
0: No response to painful stimulation	8: Unresponsive to external stimuli, including pain

Adapted from Sheahan CG, Mathews DM. Monitoring and delivery of sedation. Br J Anaesth 2014;113(Suppl 2):ii39; with permission.

The data, however, on both BIS accuracy as well as clinical utility in gastrointestinal endoscopy are conflicting. Bower and colleagues[40] found that BIS monitoring correlated well with the Observer's Assessment of Alertness/Sedation (OAA/S) across several endoscopic procedures, including EUS, ERCP, and colonoscopy (r = 0.59, $P<.0001$). In contrast, Qadeer and colleagues[41] found low accuracy of BIS in detecting deep sedation when compared with the modified OAA/S (MOAA/S) as a reference standard. There are numerous studies showing that BIS monitoring improves propofol titration and shortens recovery time,[42–45] whereas others have found no difference in these outcomes.[46–48] In 2015, Park and colleagues[49] conducted a meta analysis of 11 randomized controlled trials to address this uncertainty. With a pooled sample size of 1039 patients, they found that BIS monitoring reduced total propofol consumption (standardized mean difference −0.15, 95% confidence interval [CI] −0.28 to −0.01). There was, however, no difference in procedure time, recovery time, adverse events, or satisfaction-related outcomes. The clinical and economic value of BIS monitoring in endoscopic sedation remains controversial, and to date there is no formal recommendation on this subject from the ASA or ASGE.

ALTERNATIVE AND EMERGING TECHNIQUES

Several techniques have garnered ongoing interest in the effort to improve monitoring during endoscopic sedation. Devices designed to improve ventilation assessment include transcutaneous CO_2 monitors, respiratory volume monitors, and acoustic respiratory rate (RR) monitors. Novel techniques to evaluate depth of sedation include auditory evoked potential (AEP) monitors and functional near-infrared spectroscopy. The evidence base for all of these approaches is limited or evolving, and as of this writing there are no formal recommendations for or against their use.

Transcutaneous Carbon Dioxide Monitoring

Transcutaneous CO_2 monitors use a glass electrode to measure pH changes resulting from CO_2 diffusion across the skin. This value reflects arterial Pco_2 levels. Nelson and colleagues[50] randomized 395 patients undergoing ERCP to transcutaneous CO_2 monitoring or not and found that the intervention arm had fewer episodes of severe hypercarbia (0 of 199 vs 5 of 196, $P = .03$) and less procedural discomfort (8.3% vs 11.5%, $P = .04$). Transcutaneous monitors, however, are less effective in detecting apneas than conventional capnography[51]; their use in gastrointestinal endoscopy has been limited.

Respiratory Volume Monitors

A novel respiratory volume monitor (RVM) has been developed to tightly monitor ventilation in nonintubated patients. This technology operates by detecting thoracic impedance through electrodes placed over the patients' chest, enabling real-time calculations of RR, tidal volume (TV), and minute ventilation (MV). The RVM was designed to address well-described shortcomings in capnography, including inaccuracies with improper sensor placement, TV variation, and gas flow rate.[52–54] Voscopoulos and colleagues[55] demonstrated that the RVM is accurate in determining RR, TV, and MV as compared with spirometry as a gold standard. Holley and colleagues[56] thereafter tested RVMs in patients undergoing upper endoscopy, finding that it was highly accurate in detecting hypoventilation, even when diminished RR was not present. Further studies and head-to-head trials are needed to determine the applicability of RVMs in endoscopic sedation.

Acoustic Monitoring

Acoustic RR monitors (RRa) are a new technology that measures RR through an audio sensor placed over the neck that detects breath sounds. In 2013 Goudra and colleagues[57] compared RRa with capnography and RVM usage in patients undergoing upper endoscopy with propofol sedation. They found that RRa monitoring had comparable or improved sensitivity and specificity for apnea events (73% and 93%, respectively) as compared with RVM (45% and 93%) and capnography (73% and 12%). Tanaka and colleagues[58] found RRa to have a higher positive likelihood ratio of detecting respiratory pauses when compared with capnography or clinician observation in patients undergoing monitored anesthesia care (4.1 vs 1.0 vs 3.5, respectively). Based on these studies, acoustic monitoring may reduce false-positive alarms as compared with capnography and warrants further evaluation.

Auditory Evoked Potentials

Given the conflicting evidence base described earlier for BIS monitoring, alternative EEG-based indices have emerged. AEPs are EEG changes provoked by auditory stimuli. AEP monitors generate data that can be consolidated into a sedation index, called the A-line AEP index (AAI). Although early data show that AAI correlates well with OAA/S scoring ($\rho = 0.886$, $P<.001$),[59] head-to-head studies suggest that AAI has poorer performance characteristics as compared with BIS.[60,61] Future iterations and refinements of EEG-based methods are likely to emerge, as there remains great interest in noninvasive and accurate monitors of anesthetic depth.

Functional Near-Infrared Spectroscopy

BIS and AAI indices correlate with sedation scoring scales but do not discriminate well between sedation stages.[61] Functional near-infrared spectroscopy (fNIRS) is a noninvasive neuroimaging modality used to detect changes in cortical blood hemoglobin oxygenation.[62] These changes correlate with neuronal activity and may provide information regarding depth of sedation. In 2014 Curtin and colleagues[63] monitored 41 patients undergoing colonoscopy with fNIRS and showed that hemoglobin oxygenation in the dorsolateral prefrontal cortex correlated with changes in proposal boluses and infusions. fNIRS is an active area of investigation, and future studies are needed to define a sedation index and compare it with existing reference standards in a controlled fashion.

SUMMARY

Unplanned cardiopulmonary complications occur in 0.9% of gastrointestinal endoscopies overall, or 1 in 111 cases, when intravenous sedation is used. Complicated procedures, such as ERCP, may have rates as high as 2.1%, or 1 in 48 cases.[5] Recommended monitoring practices are designed to prevent these complications through minimization of anesthetic dosing and early detection of oversedation. Although the supporting evidence is limited, it is nearly universally accepted that close patient monitoring through visual assessment and physiologic parameters will minimize sedation-related complications. Furthermore, patients who are high risk or require deeper levels of sedation for complicated procedures warrant more intensive monitoring, including continuous electrocardiography and capnography. Devices, however, are not a replacement for skilled personnel who are able to recognize developing complications at an early stage and promptly initiate corrective management.[21] Ultimately, improved patient safety with endoscopic sedation will hinge on a combination of effective monitoring technologies and staff who are not only well trained in their use but also in attentive direct assessment of patients.

ACKNOWLEDGMENTS

The authors would like to thank Dr Sheila Barnett for critical review of this article.

REFERENCES

1. Radaelli F, Meucci G, Sgroi G, et al. Technical performance of colonoscopy: the key role of sedation/analgesia and other quality indicators. Am J Gastroenterol 2008;103(5):1122–30.
2. Cohen LB, Wecsler JS, Gaetano JN, et al. Endoscopic sedation in the United States: results from a nationwide survey. Am J Gastroenterol 2006;101(5):967–74.
3. Green SM, Mason KP. Reformulation of the sedation continuum. JAMA 2010; 303(9):876–7.
4. American Society of Anesthesiologists Task Force on Sedation and Analgesia by Non-Anesthesiologists. Practice guidelines for sedation and analgesia by non-anesthesiologists. Anesthesiology 2002;96(4):1004–17.
5. Sharma VK, Nguyen CC, Crowell MD, et al. A national study of cardiopulmonary unplanned events after GI endoscopy. Gastrointest Endosc 2007;66(1):27–34.
6. Waring JP, Baron TH, Hirota WK, et al. Guidelines for conscious sedation and monitoring during gastrointestinal endoscopy. Gastrointest Endosc 2003;58(3): 317–22.
7. Joint Commission on Accreditation of Healthcare Organizations. Standards for ambulatory care. Oakbrook Terrace (IL): Joint Commission Resources; 2009.
8. Jain R, Ikenberry SO, Anderson MA, et al. Minimum staffing requirements for the performance of GI endoscopy. Gastrointest Endosc 2010;72(3):469–70.
9. Lichtenstein DR, Jagannath S, Baron TH, et al. Sedation and anesthesia in GI endoscopy. Gastrointest Endosc 2008;68(5):815–26.
10. Cohen LB, Delegge MH, Aisenberg J, et al. AGA Institute review of endoscopic sedation. Gastroenterology 2007;133(2):675–701.
11. DiSario JA, Waring JP, Talbert G, et al. Monitoring of blood pressure and heart rate during routine endoscopy: a prospective, randomized, controlled study. Am J Gastroenterol 1991;86(8):956–60.
12. Calderwood AH, Chapman FJ, Cohen J, et al. Guidelines for safety in the gastro-intestinal endoscopy unit. Gastrointest Endosc 2014;79(3):363–72.
13. Standards for basic anesthetic monitoring. 2015. Available at: http://www.asahq.org/~/media/Sites/ASAHQ/Files/Public/Resources/standards-guidelines/standards-for-basic-anesthetic-monitoring.pdf. Accessed December 31, 2015.
14. Godwin SA, Caro DA, Wolf SJ, et al. Clinical policy: procedural sedation and anal-gesia in the emergency department. Ann Emerg Med 2005;45(2):177–96.
15. The use of pulse oximetry during conscious sedation. Council on Scientific Affairs, American Medical Association. JAMA 1993;270(12):1463–8.
16. Fu ES, Downs JB, Schweiger JW, et al. Supplemental oxygen impairs detection of hypoventilation by pulse oximetry. Chest J 2004;126(5):1552–8.
17. Hamber EA, Bailey PL, James SW, et al. Delays in the detection of hypoxemia due to site of pulse oximetry probe placement. J Clin Anesth 1999;11(2):113–8.
18. Jubran A. Pulse oximetry. Intensive Care Med 2004;30(11):2017–20.
19. Moller JT, Johannessen NW, Espersen K, et al. Randomized evaluation of pulse oximetry in 20,802 patients: II. Perioperative events and postoperative complications. Anesthesiology 1993;78(3):445–53.

20. Pedersen T, Nicholson A, Hovhannisyan K, et al. Pulse oximetry for perioperative monitoring. Cochrane Database Syst Rev 2014;(3):CD002013.

21. Cohen LB. Patient monitoring during gastrointestinal endoscopy: why, when, and how? Gastrointest Endosc Clin N Am 2008;18(4):651–63.

22. Arakawa H, Kaise M, Sumiyama K, et al. Does pulse oximetry accurately monitor a patient's ventilation during sedated endoscopy under oxygen supplementation? Singapore Med J 2013;54(4):212–5.

23. Eisenach JC. Capnography. J Am Soc Anesthesiologists 2001;95(4):1049.

24. Pekdemir M, Cinar O, Yilmaz S, et al. Disparity between mainstream and sidestream end-tidal carbon dioxide values and arterial carbon dioxide levels. Respir Care 2013;58(7):1152–6.

25. Poirier MP, Del-Rey JAG, McAneney CM, et al. Utility of monitoring capnography, pulse oximetry, and vital signs in the detection of airway mishaps: a hyperoxemic animal model. Am J Emerg Med 1998;16(4):350–2.

26. Vargo JJ, Zuccaro G, Dumot JA, et al. Automated graphic assessment of respiratory activity is superior to pulse oximetry and visual assessment for the detection of early respiratory depression during therapeutic upper endoscopy. Gastrointest Endosc 2002;55(7):826–31.

27. Radaelli F, Terruzzi V, Minoli G. Extended/advanced monitoring techniques in gastrointestinal endoscopy. Gastrointest Endosc Clin N Am 2004;14(2):335–52.

28. Cacho G, Perez-Calle JL, Barbado A, et al. Capnography is superior to pulse oximetry for the detection of respiratory depression during colonoscopy. Rev Esp Enferm Dig 2010;102(2):86–9.

29. Waugh JB, Epps CA, Khodneva YA. Capnography enhances surveillance of respiratory events during procedural sedation: a meta-analysis. J Clin Anesth 2011; 23(3):189–96.

30. Qadeer MA, Vargo JJ, Dumot JA, et al. Capnographic monitoring of respiratory activity improves safety of sedation for endoscopic cholangiopancreatography and ultrasonography. Gastroenterology 2009;136(5):1568–76 [quiz: 1819–20].

31. Beitz A, Riphaus A, Meining A, et al. Capnographic monitoring reduces the incidence of arterial oxygen desaturation and hypoxemia during propofol sedation for colonoscopy: a randomized, controlled study (ColoCap Study). Am J Gastroenterol 2012;107(8):1205–12.

32. Lightdale JR, Goldmann DA, Feldman HA, et al. Microstream capnography improves patient monitoring during moderate sedation: a randomized, controlled trial. Pediatrics 2006;117(6):e1170–8.

33. Koniaris LG, Wilson S, Drugas G, et al. Capnographic monitoring of ventilatory status during moderate (conscious) sedation. Surg Endosc 2003;17(8):1261–5.

34. Vargo JJ, Cohen LB, Rex DK, et al. Position statement: nonanesthesiologist administration of propofol for GI endoscopy. Gastrointest Endosc 2009;70(6): 1053–9.

35. Endoscopy ASfG. American College of Gastroenterology. Statement: universal adoption of capnography for moderate sedation in adults undergoing upper endoscopy and colonoscopy has not been shown to improve patient safety or clinical outcomes and significantly increases costs for moderate sedation. 2012. Available at: http://www.asge.org/WorkArea/showcontent.aspx?id=14226. Accessed March 19, 2016.

36. Weaver J. The latest ASA mandate: CO2 monitoring for moderate and deep sedation. Anesth Prog 2011;58(3):111–2.

37. Kowalski R, Mahon P, Boylan G, et al. Validity of the modified observer's assessment of alertness/sedation scale (MOAA/S) during low dose propofol sedation: 3AP6-3. Eur J Anaesthesiol 2007;24:26–7.

38. Gill M, Green SM, Krauss B. A study of the bispectral index monitor during procedural sedation and analgesia in the emergency department. Ann Emerg Med 2003;41(2):234–41.

39. Rosow C, Manberg PJ. Bispectral index monitoring. Anesthesiol Clin North America 2001;19(4):947–66, xi.

40. Bower AL, Ripepi A, Dilger J, et al. Bispectral index monitoring of sedation during endoscopy. Gastrointest Endosc 2000;52(2):192–6.

41. Qadeer MA, Vargo JJ, Patel S, et al. Bispectral index monitoring of conscious sedation with the combination of meperidine and midazolam during endoscopy. Clin Gastroenterol Hepatol 2008;6(1):102–8.

42. Wehrmann T, Grotkamp J, Stergiou N, et al. Electroencephalogram monitoring facilitates sedation with propofol for routine ERCP: a randomized, controlled trial. Gastrointest Endosc 2002;56(6):817–24.

43. Bell J, Laasch H-U, Wilbraham L, et al. Bispectral index monitoring for conscious sedation in intervention: better, safer, faster. Clin Radiol 2004;59(12):1106–13.

44. Paspatis G, Chainaki I, Manolaraki M, et al. Efficacy of bispectral index monitoring as an adjunct to propofol deep sedation for ERCP: a randomized controlled trial. Endoscopy 2009;41(12):1046.

45. Von Delius S, Salletmaier H, Meining A, et al. Bispectral index monitoring of midazolam and propofol sedation during endoscopic retrograde cholangiopancreatography: a randomized clinical trial (the EndoBIS study). Endoscopy 2012;44(3):258–64.

46. Drake LM, Chen SC, Rex DK. Efficacy of bispectral monitoring as an adjunct to nurse-administered propofol sedation for colonoscopy: a randomized controlled trial. Am J Gastroenterol 2006;101(9):2003–7.

47. DeWitt JM. Bispectral index monitoring for nurse-administered propofol sedation during upper endoscopic ultrasound: a prospective, randomized controlled trial. Dig Dis Sci 2008;53(10):2739–45.

48. Imagawa A, Fujiki S, Kawahara Y, et al. Satisfaction with bispectral index monitoring of propofol-mediated sedation during endoscopic submucosal dissection: a prospective, randomized study. Endoscopy 2008;40(11):905–9.

49. Park SW, Lee H, Ahn H. Bispectral index versus standard monitoring in sedation for endoscopic procedures: a systematic review and meta-analysis. Dig Dis Sci 2016;61(3):814–24.

50. Nelson DB, Freeman ML, Silvis SE, et al. A randomized, controlled trial of transcutaneous carbon dioxide monitoring during ERCP. Gastrointest Endosc 2000;51(3):288–95.

51. De Oliveira G, Ahmad S, Fitzgerald P, et al. Detection of hypoventilation during deep sedation in patients undergoing ambulatory gynaecological hysteroscopy: a comparison between transcutaneous and nasal end-tidal carbon dioxide measurements. Br J Anaesth 2010;104(6):774–8.

52. Bhananker SM, Posner KL, Cheney FW, et al. Injury and liability associated with monitored anesthesia care a closed claims analysis. J Am Soc Anesthesiologists 2006;104(2):228–34.

53. Jabre P, Jacob L, Auger H, et al. Capnography monitoring in nonintubated patients with respiratory distress. Am J Emerg Med 2009;27(9):1056–9.

54. van Loon K, van Rheineck Leyssius AT, van Zaane B, et al. Capnography during deep sedation with propofol by nonanesthesiologists: a randomized controlled trial. Anesth Analg 2014;119(1):49–55.
55. Voscopoulos C, Brayanov J, Ladd D, et al. Evaluation of a novel noninvasive respiration monitor providing continuous measurement of minute ventilation in ambulatory subjects in a variety of clinical scenarios. Anesth Analg 2013; 117(1):91–100.
56. Holley K, MacNabb CM, Georgiadis P, et al. Monitoring minute ventilation versus respiratory rate to measure the adequacy of ventilation in patients undergoing upper endoscopic procedures. J Clin Monit Comput 2016;30(1):33–9.
57. Goudra BG, Penugonda LC, Speck RM. Comparison of acoustic respiration rate, impedance pneumography and capnometry monitors for respiration rate accuracy and apnea detection during GI endoscopy anesthesia. Open Journal of Anesthesiology 2013;3:74–9.
58. Tanaka PP, Tanaka M, Drover DR. Detection of respiratory compromise by acoustic monitoring, capnography, and brain function monitoring during monitored anesthesia care. J Clin Monit Comput 2014;28(6):561–6.
59. Huang Y-Y, Chu Y-C, Chang K-Y, et al. Performance of AEP monitor/2-derived composite index as an indicator for depth of sedation with midazolam and alfentanil during gastrointestinal endoscopy. Eur J Anaesthesiol 2007;24(3):252–7.
60. Struys M, Jensen EW, Smith W, et al. Performance of the ARX-derived auditory evoked potential index as an indicator of anesthetic depth: a comparison with bispectral index and hemodynamic measures during propofol administration. Anesthesiology 2002;96(4):803–16.
61. von Delius S, Thies P, Rieder T, et al. Auditory evoked potentials compared with bispectral index for monitoring of midazolam and propofol sedation during colonoscopy. Am J Gastroenterol 2009;104(2):318–25.
62. Wolf M, Ferrari M, Quaresima V. Progress of near-infrared spectroscopy and topography for brain and muscle clinical applications. J Biomed Opt 2007; 12(6):062104.
63. Curtin A, Izzetoglu K, Reynolds J, et al. Functional near-infrared spectroscopy for the measurement of propofol effects in conscious sedation during outpatient elective colonoscopy. Neuroimage 2014;85:626–36.

Sedation and Monitoring in the Pediatric Patient during Gastrointestinal Endoscopy

Hyun Kee Chung, MD[a], Jenifer R. Lightdale, MD, MPH[b],*

KEYWORDS

- Sedation • Pediatrics • Procedural sedation • General anesthesia • Sedatives
- Endoscopy • Gastrointestinal • Gastrointestinal procedures

KEY POINTS

- To date, there is no single sedative or combined regimen that has been established as ideal for pediatric gastrointestinal (GI) procedures, regardless of whether procedural sedation is administered by endoscopists or anesthesiologists.
- Over the past decade, more pediatric endoscopy is being performed with anesthesiologist-administered sedation, specifically with propofol.
- Broadly speaking, sedation plans that call for general anesthesia with endotracheal intubation are not necessary for routine pediatric endoscopy or colonoscopy and may decrease procedural efficiency and value.
- It is becoming increasingly important for pediatric endoscopists to engage in a dialogue with anesthesiologists, with the goal of determining best sedation practices for children undergoing GI procedures.

INTRODUCTION

The role of endoscopy in the diagnosis and treatment of digestive diseases of childhood has grown steadily over the past 40 years. In turn, the need to identify best practices for sedating children undergoing GI procedures has intensified. Generally speaking, the provision of sedation for endoscopy is considered necessary if children are to remain safe, comfortable, and cooperative. Nevertheless, no single sedative or combined sedation regimen has yet been established as ideal for pediatric GI procedures.

Conflict of Interest Statement: Medtronic (consultant), Mead-Johnson (speaker), Perrigo (advisory board) (J.R. Lightdale). None (H.K. Chung).
[a] Pediatric Anesthesia, Department of Anesthesia, UMass Memorial Medical Center, 55 Lake Street North, Worcester, MA 01655, USA; [b] Pediatric Gastroenterology and Nutrition, UMass Memorial Children's Medical Center, University Campus, 55 Lake Street North, Worcester, MA 01655, USA
* Corresponding author.
E-mail address: jenifer.lightdale@umassmemorial.org

Gastrointest Endoscopy Clin N Am 26 (2016) 507–525
http://dx.doi.org/10.1016/j.giec.2016.02.004
1052-5157/16/$ – see front matter © 2016 Elsevier Inc. All rights reserved.

giendo.theclinics.com

Over the past 10 years, a considerable change in the landscape of sedation practices has occurred, with more and more pediatric endoscopy performed in the presence of anesthesiology providers. Although a 2005 survey of members of the North American Society of Pediatric Gastroenterology, Hepatology and Nutrition suggested wide practice variation in types of sedation at that time,[1] more recent data suggest that anesthesiologist-administered sedation, specifically with propofol, is becoming the more common experience.[2] In turn, it is becoming imperative that anesthesiologists gain knowledge about various pediatric endoscopic procedures as well as evolving evidence for best sedation practices. At the same time, it remains incumbent on endoscopists who perform procedures in children to be knowledgeable about sedation as well as to maintain familiarity with its various educational curricula and guidelines.[3]

Generally speaking, most procedural sedation for pediatric endoscopy involves intravenous (IV) medications and ideally maintains a child's ability to breathe spontaneously with intact protective airway reflexes. Procedural sedation for pediatric endoscopy may be administered by an anesthesiologist or by an endoscopist in the absence of an anesthesiologist. When an anesthesiologist is involved, it may be acceptable to aim for deep levels of sedation that may verge into general anesthesia.[4] In the absence of an anesthesiologist, it is important that endoscopists are familiar with regimens effective at achieving moderate sedation and know how to rescue patients should the level of sedation become deeper than expected.[3]

Given that many children undergoing stressful and uncomfortable procedures may be agitated,[5] it is becoming more common to plan for deep levels of sedation for pediatric patients undergoing diagnostic endoscopy.[6] Another primary option for endoscopic sedation in children is general anesthesia with inhalational anesthetics, often in combination with IV agents. Broadly speaking, sedation plans that call for general anesthesia with endotracheal intubation are not necessary for routine pediatric endoscopic procedures. Instead, protocols that seek to achieve general anesthetic sedation levels necessitating endotracheal intubation can be reserved for therapeutic cases as well as endoscopy in very young or medically complex patients.

One important factor driving changes in sedation practices for pediatric endoscopy may be the need to identify means of improving efficiency.[7] In addition, there is increasing pressure to reduce costs.[8] To this end, using anesthesiologists, especially in operating room settings, for brief procedures that do not require patients to be fully immobile may involve excessive use of health care resources.[2,8,9] Although only 10% of respondents in 2005 reported using general anesthesia for all procedures, a full third reported mostly performing procedures with general anesthesia in hospital operating rooms.[1] Another third of respondents reported performing more than three-quarters of their procedures with anesthesiologist-administered propofol in a dedicated endoscopy facility, outside of main operating rooms. Today, the performance of pediatric endoscopy outside of the main operating room has become standard practice.[2,6]

Patient safety should and does remain paramount. In this regard, it has become clear that the use of procedural sedation to achieve all levels of consciousness (moderate, deep, and general anesthesia) represents the most common risk factor for endoscopy complications.[2,7,10] Complications due to sedation, regardless of who has administered it, have been consistently documented to occur more commonly during pediatric endoscopy than technical complications related to procedures, such as bleeding or perforation.[11–14] As such, the intersection between performance of GI procedures in children, efficiency, costs, patient safety, and sedation has remained a topic of great interest among pediatric gastroenterologists for the past 4 decades.[9,11,15] It is also gaining interest in the world of anesthesiologists, who are increasingly recognizing that best approaches for sedating children for pediatric endoscopy may be quite different from those of other pediatric procedures as well as from sedation of adults for GI procedures.[10]

In short, all endoscopists, whether or not they work with anesthesiologists, should understand the myriad implications of sedation choices inherent to performing GI procedures in children.[3,6] Those endoscopists who work with anesthesiologists, including pediatric gastroenterologists who do this exclusively, should also have a working knowledge of approaches that anesthesiologists may use to achieve procedural sedation. **Box 1** lists several patient risk factors for complications during

---

Box 1
Patient risk factors for sedation/anesthesia complications during pediatric gastrointestinal procedures

- Patient age

- Planned procedure

- Concerns for high body mass index

- Relevant comorbidities
  - Anxiety
  - Cardiac disease
  - Diabetes
  - Reactive airways
  - Seizure disorder
  - Psychiatric disorders

- Aspiration risk factors
  - Achalasia
  - Emergency procedures
  - Food/foreign body impaction
  - Full-column gastroesophageal reflux (by clinical history)

- Concerns for difficult airways
  - Congenital abnormalities
    - Pierre Robin syndrome
    - Treacher Collins syndrome
    - Laryngeal atresia
    - Craniofacial abnormalities
  - Anatomic variations
    - Large tongue
    - Highly arched or narrow palate
    - Short, thick neck
    - Prominent overbite
    - Limited range of motion of neck

- Relevant medications
  - Cardiopulmonary
  - Antiseizure
  - Psychotropic
  - Analgesics
    - Benzodiazepines
    - Opioids

- History of recreational drug use

- Known social considerations
  - Limitations of parental presence/right to consent
  - Legal guardian information

Consideration of these factors and others should be communicated prior to the procedure by endoscopists to all providers, including anesthesiologists, involved in administering sedation.

procedural sedation and anesthesia that should be discussed by endoscopists working with anesthesiologists to perform sedated endoscopy in children.

This article reviews a broad clinical experience with traditional and newer sedatives for pediatric GI endoscopy, with a focus on benefits, limitations, and pitfalls of various regimens.[16–19] Both traditional and innovative sedative regimens are discussed as well as opportunities for minimizing patient risk while optimizing procedural efficiency. The importance of engaging in a dialogue with pediatric anesthesiologists, who are increasingly called on to gain familiarity with best practices for sedating children to undergo pediatric endoscopy, is also emphasized.

GOALS AND LEVELS OF SEDATION FOR PEDIATRIC GASTROINTESTINAL PROCEDURES

The primary purpose of sedation for children undergoing upper and lower endoscopies is to perform procedures safely, with a minimal amount of emotional and physical discomfort. Secondary and often desirable goals of sedation are to affect periprocedural amnesia, maximize procedural efficiency, minimize recovery times, and maintain cost effectiveness. Although some GI procedures may be preferentially performed without sedation, almost all require some sedative regimen to ensure patient cooperation. Historically, gastroenterologists have measured sedation success using several different benchmarks (**Box 2**). To objectively compare regimens, it may be preferable to use independent observers and standardized scales.[7,20]

In terms of the levels of sedation that can be achieved, there are 4 that have been defined to stretch along a continuum without clear boundaries: minimal, moderate, deep, and general anesthesia.[21] These levels are defined by a patient's response to verbal, light tactile, or painful stimuli and are generally also associated with physiologic changes in patient vital signs. Minimal sedation implies the retention of a patient's ability to respond voluntarily to vocal commands (eg, "take a deep breath" or "turn on your back") and to maintain a patent airway with protective reflexes. Moderate sedation describes a depth of sedation at which patients are able to tolerate unpleasant procedures while maintaining adequate cardiorespiratory function, protective airway reflexes, and the ability to react to verbal or tactile stimulation. Deep sedation implies a medically controlled state of depressed consciousness from which a patient is not easily aroused but may respond purposefully to painful stimulation. General

---

Box 2
Parameters that can be used to assess sedation regimens for pediatric endoscopy

Sedation measures

- Adverse events related to sedation
- Adverse events related to procedure
- Procedure completion rate
- Procedure times
- Patient recovery times
- Patient satisfaction
- Provider satisfaction
- Cost
- Speed of recovery of cognition
- Speed of recovery of locomotion

anesthesia describes the deepest level of sedation where a patient is unconscious, with reduced responses to stimuli and with an airway that may require support.

Optimal levels of sedation may vary depending on the procedure. In upper endoscopy, a major goal of sedation may be to avoid gagging and increase patient cooperation; in colonoscopy, the goal of sedation is often to avoid visceral pain associated with looping. Child anxiety levels may also vary for different procedures and may be mediated by other practice choices. For upper endoscopy, both premedication with topical sprays and premedication with oral sedatives prior to IV line insertion have been shown to independently improve pediatric patient tolerance and satisfaction.[22,23]

Generally speaking, depth of sedation is directly related to cardiovascular stability; the deeper the level of sedation, the more a patient is considered at risk for cardiopulmonary events (**Fig. 1**). During all sedated GI procedures, even those conducted with anesthesiologist assistance, pediatric endoscopists must be exquisitely familiar with the fine line between achieving adequate light sedation and creating the potential for a child to become deeply sedated.[24] For instance, deep sedation may develop in lightly sedated patients due to delayed drug absorption or a secondary decrease in painful stimuli common to procedures (eg, after successful navigation of the hepatic flexure during pediatric colonoscopy).[25,26]

Over the past decade, it has become standard to work with an anesthesiologist to achieve deep sedation verging into general anesthesia.[27] To some extent, this is the most reliable level of sedation to plan for in children to assure tolerance of the procedure without signs of distress that may include vocalization and disruptive movements. Many endoscopists who previously may have performed procedures with endoscopist-administered moderate sedation, and who have had experience with children struggling throughout procedures, have recognized the benefits of being assured that a child is deeply sedated for the procedure. In turn, there has been a strong movement toward increased use of anesthesiologist-administered sedation in pediatric endoscopy.

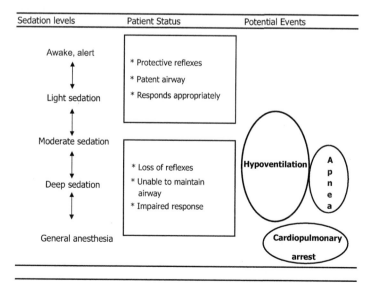

Fig. 1. Commonly used terms to describe sedation, their relationship to the continuum of sedation levels, and their relationship to potential adverse events.

UNSEDATED PROCEDURES

Recently, unsedated transnasal endoscopy has been investigated as a safe and effective means of monitoring the esophageal mucosa of pediatric patients with eosinophilic esophagitis.[28] In such procedures, very-small-diameter (ie, 2.8–4 mm) scopes are used in the office, with a reported high patient satisfaction score. Further studies are needed to determine whether such protocols are generalizable to other centers but hold promise that certain pediatric endoscopic procedures someday may be performed without sedation.

In the meantime, it is true that it remains possible to perform standard upper and lower endoscopic procedures in infants and small children without sedation, especially if they are restrained.[29] The routine use of this method is not recommended and may be considered unethical when there are safe forms of IV sedation or general anesthesia available.[30–32] In turn, the practice of performing endoscopic procedures in children without sedation seems to be falling out of favor with most contemporary pediatric GI practitioners, especially as greater access to anesthesiologists has become standard in the majority of endoscopy units worldwide.[9]

PATIENT RISK STRATIFICATION AND AIRWAY ASSESSMENT

Sedation for pediatric GI procedures should be tailored to a patient's physical status, in accordance with guidelines from the American Society of Anesthesiologists (**Table 1**).[33] Taking into account a patient's age and developmental status when choosing a sedation regimen may also improve procedural success. Data suggest that the smallest and youngest pediatric patients with the highest American Society of Anesthesiologists classifications are at greatest risk for complications during GI procedures.[10,13]

Personality and psychosocial development stages may vary widely among children undergoing GI procedures, which may have a great impact on their reactions to sedatives in terms of both rapidity and depth of sedation achieved.[30,34] Patients can be approximately classified as less than 6 months, greater than 6 months, school aged (4–11 years), and adolescents. Infants under 6 months of age may have little anxiety and tend to sedate easily. Infants greater than 6 months who have developed stranger anxiety may more smoothly sedate if parents remain next to them during induction. School-aged children manifest concrete thinking and may be surprisingly difficult to sedate, belying higher anxiety levels than may be appreciated.[35] Adolescents may be composed during preprocedure preparations and then become disinhibited and exhibit strong anxiety with initial doses of sedatives.

Table 1	
American Society of Anesthesiologists classification of patients' physical status	
American Society of Anesthesiologists Class	**Physical Status**
1	Normal healthy patient
2	Patient with mild systemic disease
3	Patient with severe systemic disease
4	Patient with severe systemic disease that is a constant threat to life
5	Moribund patient not expected to survive without emergent procedure

Data from Sidi A, Lobato EB, Cohen JA. The American society of Anesthesiologists' physical status: category V revisited. J Clin Anesth 2000;12:328–34.

Especially in school-aged children, a careful discussion of what to expect during the procedure delivered in a relaxed reassuring manner may decrease patient anxiety levels.[34] Information should be imparted early in the process and include explanations about IV line insertions. Children with greater distress during the IV insertion have been shown to experience significantly greater distress and pain throughout the rest of the procedure.[36] In turn, the use of topical anesthetics for IV catheter insertion, such as topical lidocaine cream, or oral anxiolytics, such as midazolam, may be warranted.[23,36]

Regardless of sedation regimens used, it is also essential to perform airway assessments. Attention to patients' potential risk due to their airway should be paid at the time of scheduling a procedure and while performing it. Among both gastroenterologists and anesthesiologists, there is increasing interest in using grading systems, such as the Mallampati score, to assess airway risk in a standardized fashion within their unit (**Box 3**).

In deciding whether children are appropriate for endoscopist-administered procedural sedation, or even anesthesiologist-administered sedation outside the main operating room, there may be different thresholds of airway status appropriateness for management at particular facilities, depending on location and available resources.[9] To a certain extent, it may be prudent for ambulatory endoscopy centers to have stricter patient and airway criteria than academic or community hospitals, where emergency resources may be timelier in their arrival. Some GI disorders increase the riskiness of the procedure. In particular, upper GI bleeds, anatomic or physiologic obstruction of the upper GI tract, recent ingestion of blood or food, and sepsis-related biliary obstruction all place a patient at higher risk for complications both from the procedures and from the sedation.[37] In addition, premature infants as well as older children with body mass indices for age greater than the 85th percentile also may be at increased risk.

PATIENT POSITIONING

All patients undergoing diagnostic upper and lower endoscopic procedures with sedation should be placed in the left lateral decubitus position. This is because patients who are placed in the supine position are more susceptible to pooling of secretions in oral pharynx and risk upper airway obstruction or laryngospasm. Patients undergoing endoscopic retrograde cholangiopancreatography may require the prone or prone-oblique position. Airway monitoring and management are more challenging in the prone position and may require advanced monitoring.

USE OF A LARYNGEAL MASK AIRWAY

A laryngeal mask airway (LMA) is a supraglottic airway device that is positioned in the hypopharynx, providing a seal over the larynx to allow spontaneous respiration while

---

Box 3
Mallampati score for airway assessment

- Class I – uvula is completely visible
- Class II – partially visible uvula
- Class III – soft palate visible but not uvula
- Class IV – hard palate visible only, not soft or uvula

Data from Mallampati SR, Gatt SP, Gugino LD, et al. A clinical sign to predict difficult tracheal intubation: a prospective study. Can Anaesth Soc J 1985;32:429–34.

under deep sedation or general anesthesia.[38] An LMA does not protect the airway from pulmonary aspiration and is not a substitute for endotracheal intubation when indicated. Instead, an LMA is used to provide a mask general anesthetic, where the mask is applied to the laryngeal structures instead of the face. As an airway device, an LMA can be used routinely for pediatric endoscopy, especially with younger patients who may be more prone to airway obstruction.[38] An LMA is particularly compatible with diagnostic upper endoscopy in children, because small-diameter pediatric scopes can be easily passed posterior to an appropriately sized and seated LMA. Care must be taken to ensure that the LMA is not dislodged during endoscope manipulation. In addition, deeper levels of anesthesia may be required to prevent airway stimulation caused by the LMA compared with a spontaneous breathing technique. For this reason, it is not uncommon for volatile agents to be used to maintain general anesthetic levels of sedation when using the LMA.

PATIENT MONITORING

Although visual assessments are considered as important as electronic monitoring for ensuring patient safety, oxygen desaturation represents a particularly objective means of detecting poor respiratory effort in children undergoing IV sedation. Even if providers have not detected suboptimal ventilation by clinical assessment, they often intervene to stimulate patient respiration if a pulse oximeter detects minor desaturation. Oxygen desaturation is a late sign of suboptimal ventilation.[39] Patients receiving supplemental oxygen may be particularly at risk for poorly ventilating while still saturating 100% by pulse oximetry.

The dilemma posed by relying on pulse oximetry as the main means of electronically monitoring children during endoscopy is that patients may be well saturated with oxygen and simultaneously have significant carbon dioxide (CO_2) retention. Over the past decade, improved compact microstream capnographs have been developed using aspiration flow technology that allow the accurate real-time graphic display of ventilatory waveforms in nonintubated patients by measuring their end-tidal CO_2.[39,40] Using capnography in the pediatric endoscopy setting may reveal that abnormal ventilation is occurring during procedures in children at rates higher than expected.[41]

COMMON SEDATIVES USED FOR CHILDREN UNDERGOING ENDOSCOPY

There are several procedural sedation regimens that have been reported to be safe and efficacious for children undergoing procedures.[42] **Table 2** lists commonly used sedatives for pediatric GI procedures and their recommended dosages. In general, the most common procedural sedation regimens used for pediatric endoscopy combine a narcotic analgesic (eg, meperidine or fentanyl) with a benzodiazepine (eg, diazepam or midazolam), although there have been increasing reports of the use of ketamine as an alternative. Narcotics offer the benefit of analgesia. Benzodiazepines provide for anxiolysis and amnesia. Ketamine is reliable at rendering patients immobile, and mute, but they may retain awareness of the procedure.[20] Most deep sedation regimens and general anesthesia for endoscopy currently use propofol as a mainstay sedative. Propofol is an ultra–short-acting anesthetic that can be used to induce and maintain a spectrum of sedation levels, ranging from moderate sedation to general anesthesia.

Table 3 lists several drug-specific side effects associated with various sedatives and rescue agents. In addition, it is imperative that pediatric endoscopists respect the potential for oversedation regardless of regimen used and its risks of morbidity

Table 2
Recommendations for dosages of drugs commonly used for intravenous sedation for pediatric gastrointestinal procedures, including reversal agents for benzodiazepines and opioids

Sedatives	Route	Maximum Dose (mg/kg)	Time to Onset (min)	Duration of Action (min)
Benzodiazepines				
Diazepam	IV	0.1–0.3	1–3	15–30
	Rectal	0.2–0.3	2–10	15–30
Midazolam	Oral	0.5–0.75	15–30	60–90
	IV	0.05–0.15	2–3	45–60
	Rectal	0.5–0.75	10–30	60–90
Opioids				
Meperidine	IV	1–3	<5	2–4
	IM	1–3	10–15	2–3
Fentanyl	IV	0.001–0.005 (1–5 µg/kg in 0.5–1.0 µg/kg increments)	2–3	30–60
Ketamine	IV	1–3	1	15–60
	IM	2–10	3–5	15–150

Reversal Agents	Route	Maximum Dose (mg/kg)	Time to Onset (min)	Duration of Action (min)
For benzodiazepines				
Flumazenil	IV	3 mg/h	1–2	<60
For opioids				
Naloxone	IV	0.1	2–5	20–60
	IM	0.1	2–5	20–60

Table 3
Common agents for procedural sedation in endoscopy and their side effects

Class/Name	Potential Side Effects/Complications
Topical	
Benzocaine	Methemoglobinemia
Lidocaine	Potential for systemic absorption and toxicity
Benzodiazepines	
Diazepam	Respiratory depression; apnea; thrombophlebitis
Midazolam	Respiratory depression; apnea
Opioids	
Meperidine	Respiratory and central nervous system depression; seizures, nausea; vomiting
Fentanyl	Apnea, bradycardia; chest wall and glottic rigidity
Ketamine	Emergence delirium; laryngospasm
Propofol	Rapid progression to general anesthesia; impaired GI contractility
Antagonists	
Flumazenil	Short duration of action; resedation
Naloxone	Catecholamine release, tachyarrhythmias, sudden death

and mortality. In particular, it is key to understand that all sedatives have the potential to significantly depress the central nervous system. This may compromise airway protective reflexes, increasing the risk for microaspiration and gross aspiration as well as ventilatory responses to CO_2. In turn, patients may develop apnea, which can progress to CO_2 retention and hypoxemia. Ultimately, the body may develop ischemia as well as significant cardiovascular compromise.

Fentanyl

As a fat-soluble narcotic that rapidly penetrates the blood-brain barrier, fentanyl is considerably more potent and fast acting than both morphine and meperidine. Its onset of action is approximately 30 seconds, and its opioid effects last approximately 30 to 45 minutes. Fentanyl should always be given to children via slow IV push, because its rapid administration has been associated with dangerous side effects of chest wall and glottic rigidity.[43]

Fentanyl is variably metabolized by the liver, especially in young children. Several studies have suggested that fentanyl may not represent an ideal sedative for infants. In particular, it has been associated with significant apnea in infants less than 3 months of age.[44] Also, delayed fentanyl excretion has been reported in neonates with compromised hepatic blood flow.[45] These unique pharmacokinetics of fentanyl are certainly relevant to pediatric endoscopists. In particular, fentanyl's termination of action occurs with redistribution of drug metabolites from the plasma, rather than from metabolism, causing its respiratory depressive effects to outlast its opioid effects. Therefore, fentanyl is administered most safely to children in small increments, allowing for several minutes between each dose.

Midazolam

Midazolam is 3 to 6 times more potent than diazepam, with an onset of action of 1 minute to 5 minutes and peak effect achieved at approximately 30 minutes to 1 hour. Several pharmacokinetic studies have suggested that midazolam may be metabolized and excreted more rapidly in children than in adults.[23,46,47] In addition, midazolam is unique among benzodiazepines in that its clearance seems dose related, with increased clearance with increased dosage.[48] Both metabolic facts may explain why pediatric gastroenterologists have reported the need to give larger weight-adjusted doses to their patients than adult gastroenterologists to achieve similar levels and duration of sedation.[49]

Ketamine

Ketamine is a dissociative agent that largely spares upper airway muscular tone and laryngeal reflexes and may represent an alternative to narcotics and benzodiazepines for sedating children for GI procedures. As a derivative of phencyclidine, ketamine binds to opiate receptors and rapidly induces a trancelike cataleptic condition with significant analgesia. Routes of administration can be oral or rectal but generally speaking are IV or intramuscular (IM) for endoscopy.

Ketamine is contraindicated in patients less than 3 months of age as well as those with histories of airway instability, tracheal abnormalities, active pulmonary disease, cardiovascular disease, head injury, central nervous system masses, hydrocephalus, porphyria, and thyroid disease.[50] Ketamine is also contraindicated in patients with a history of psychosis, because its traditional main drawback has been its association with hallucinogenic emergence reactions in some children. It has been suggested that these effects can be lessened by the prior administration of a short-acting benzodiazepine, such as midazolam.[51] Ketamine has also been associated with increased airway secretions and increased incidence of postoperative nausea and vomiting. This may be of greater concern for endoscopists, because ketamine has also been highly associated with laryngospasm during both upper and lower GI procedures.[8,20,51–54]

Propofol

Having a patient breathe spontaneously, without endotracheal intubation, while under a propofol-based general anesthetic, is perhaps the most common approach to sedating children for pediatric endoscopy. Propofol has been shown in multiple studies to be highly effective at inducing sedation in children who are undergoing both upper and lower endoscopy and provides excellent amnesia for the procedure.[2,55–57] It may be administered during pediatric endoscopy either as a total IV anesthetic or in combination with inhalational agents.[58]

Children who receive propofol have shorter induction times than children who received midazolam and fentanyl. Nevertheless, evidence does not show that this faster induction time leads to improved procedural efficiency in pediatric endoscopy units.[7] This lack of efficiency may be in large part secondary to indisputable variation in anesthesiology practice regarding endotracheal intubation for airway protection during propofol sedation for pediatric GI procedures. Although endotracheal intubation may be necessary during therapeutic procedures, a majority of pediatric patients do not require endotracheal intubation to perform routine diagnostic endoscopy.[2]

Indications for endotracheal intubation with administration of propofol

Determining if a patient requires endotracheal intubation is a major decision that should be made during sedation planning. Children at known risk for pulmonary aspiration, or with underlying issues that increase their risk of airway obstruction, require endotracheal intubation. Procedures that are longer and more invasive have the potential to cause greater airway stimulation and thus typically require intubation. There is no age cutoff when patients require intubation, but many practitioners routinely intubate infants and toddler-aged children to prevent airway complications. Nevertheless, it is important to recognize that it is possible, and perhaps preferable, to use a propofol-based regimen for pediatric endoscopic procedures in most pediatric patients that is intended to achieve deep levels of sedation or even general anesthesia without performing endotracheal intubation.

Propofol infusion without endotracheal intubation for pediatric endoscopy

In the authors' unit, patients receiving propofol without endotracheal intubation typically receive a mask anesthetic induction with a volatile anesthetic gas for IV catheter placement. Alternatively, if a patient has an IV catheter in situ, this obviates a mask anesthetic induction. An IV induction dose of propofol of 1 mg/kg to 2 mg/kg is then administered, followed by initiation of a propofol infusion intended to maintain anesthesia. Delivering propofol via an infusion pump is recommended to gradually attain and maintain appropriate levels of anesthesia. Generally speaking, high doses, in the range of 100 µg/kg/min to 300 µg/kg/min, are required to provide ideal conditions for endoscopic procedures in pediatric patients. Pharmacokinetic studies of children who have received propofol demonstrate that average total propofol doses per kilogram of body weight to achieve targeted plasma propofol concentrations are higher in younger children.[59,60]

An important pharmacologic disadvantage of propofol is its narrow therapeutic range, characterized by a very small difference between an ideal depth of anesthesia and respiratory depression. For this reason, providing a bolus propofol for inadequate anesthesia may result in apnea. One recent study by Kaddu and colleagues[56] reported that 20% of pediatric patients receiving anesthesiologist-administered propofol for upper endoscopy experienced transient apnea.

Once an appropriate level of anesthesia is attained, the anesthetic gas, if used, is discontinued, a nasal cannula equipped with CO_2 monitoring is taped into place, a pediatric bite block is inserted, and the patient is placed in the lateral decubitus position, as described previously. When the endoscopist introduces the endoscope, extending the patient's neck can facilitate its passage. Maintaining a manual jaw thrust during the entire procedure may be appropriate to keep the airway patent and for many anesthesiologists is a standard component of sedation for pediatric endoscopy.

Anticipatory guidance for propofol sedation for pediatric endoscopy

It is helpful to anticipate that insertion of the endoscope typically is the most stimulating part of an upper procedure. In turn, the use of local anesthetics to anesthetize the airway prior to administration of inhalational anesthetics or sedation doses of various agents, including propofol, is also recommended in patients who can tolerate the topical administration. Anesthetizing the airway has been shown to be effective at reducing the incidence of coughing and bucking during the procedure. In addition, it is the authors' experience that with less airway sensitivity, the total propofol requirement is decreased.

In the authors' protocol, 2 sprays of topical lidocaine are administered using a disposable aerosolizing device. With the patient in a sitting position, a tongue depressor is used, and the patient is instructed to phonate "ahh" to expose the posterior oral pharynx and base of the tongue. The first spray is straight back into the oral pharynx. This can cause some gagging so the patient should be allowed to recover before proceeding with the final spray. The second spray is directed 90° downward to anesthetize the hypopharynx and the glottic structures. Staying within maximal milligram/kilogram lidocaine doses and avoiding the routine use of benzocaine in children can avoid the toxicity of local anesthetics.

As another anticipatory precaution around upper endoscopic intubation, the authors also typically continue any volatile anesthetic gas that may have been used for IV line insertion for as long as possible, to ensure a patient's airway is deeply anesthetized prior to insertion of the endoscope. If the patient responds to endoscope insertion attempts with coughing and movement, the propofol infusion rate is increased by 50 µg/kg/min to 100 µg/kg/min and small bolus doses of 0.5 mg/kg are administered if required. Should apnea occur, a jaw thrust maneuver may be all that is needed to open an obstructed airway and provide enough stimulation to restore spontaneous respirations. If the patient becomes hypoxic and demonstrates significant oxygen desaturation, the endoscope should be removed, and bag mask ventilation should be provided until spontaneous respirations return.

If the patient continues to be intolerant to the spontaneously breathing technique for whatever reason, the decision can be made to place an endotracheal tube. This definitively controls the airway and allows the procedure to continue in a safe and efficient manner.

Propofol sedation for pediatric colonoscopy

A spontaneously breathing, propofol-based regimen intended to provide deep sedation verging on general anesthesia is well suited for lower endoscopic procedures.[61] In colonoscopy, the risk of airway compromise exists, but it is greatly reduced compared with upper endoscopy procedures that stimulate the airway. On the other hand, colonoscopic procedures may be more painful than upper procedures. Loop formation of the scope as well as maneuvers performed to reduce this (ie, the application of external abdominal pressure) may cause pain and patient movement, leading to increased sedation requirements.

For this reason, propofol sedation for colonoscopy generally involves use of an opioid, typically fentanyl, 0.5 μg/kg.[62] Alternatively, attempting to maintain sedation with propofol as a sole agent may require high doses to keep patients from reacting to pain. It is important for anesthesia providers to recognize potential discomfort associated with colonoscopy. Because propofol does not have analgesic properties, attempts to make a patient motionless with higher doses increase the depth of anesthesia and increase the risk of respiratory depression and apnea. A balanced sedation/anesthetic with propofol attempts to maximize the benefits of a combination of agents while minimizing the unwanted side effects of specific agents. Adding judicious amounts of a short-acting opioid should treat painful stimuli and even reduce the propofol requirement. Opioids themselves can cause hypoventilation in a dose-dependent way, but careful weight-based dosing and titration in children should result in the desired balanced effect.

Emergence from propofol sedation

It is the authors' protocol to stop the propofol infusion approximately 5 to 10 minutes before the end of a GI procedure and keep the child in the lateral decubitus position until the endoscope is withdrawn and bite block removed. With this protocol, emergence from anesthesia is not required in the procedure room, and the patient can be transported to the pediatric postanesthetic care unit (PACU) with supplemental oxygen while still asleep. This is one of the efficiency benefits of the spontaneously breathing technique; no extubation or emergence is required in the procedure room. The patient is allowed to slowly emerge from the anesthesia in PACU, which is usually much smoother than the rapid wake-ups attempted in the procedure room.

Propofol with endotracheal intubation

When patients are at risk for pulmonary aspiration, endotracheal intubation is indicated. Aspiration risk is determined by history and physical examination and may be confirmed with diagnostic studies.[37] Patients with airway abnormalities that predispose to obstruction should also have their airways secured with an endotracheal tube. Patients who require endotracheal intubation for nonaspiration reasons can be induced and intubated using standard anesthetic techniques.

Children who are clinically judged to have the potential for full-esophageal column reflux during procedural sedation, as well as those who may require procedures despite likely esophageal or gastric contents (eg, patients with achalasia or those who require emergency button-battery removal), may be appropriate candidates for a rapid sequence induction (RSI) to minimize the risk of pulmonary aspiration with the induction of general anesthesia.[63] RSI renders patients unconscious and achieves muscle relaxation with the goal of establishing ideal tracheal intubating conditions. RSI should not be used in patients who have potential difficult direct laryngoscopies (ie, Mallampati IV). Rather, other specialized intubating techniques are required for patients with the known difficult airway.

During RSI prior to GI procedures in children, propofol dosed at 2 mg/kg to 5 mg/kg represents a typical induction agent, whereas the depolarizing neuromuscular blocking agent succinylcholine, dosed at 1 mg/kg to 2 mg/kg, is used as the ideal neuromuscular blocking agent. In patients where the use of succinylcholine is contraindicated, the nondepolarizing muscle relaxant, rocuronium, can be considered a reliable alternative when given in an RSI dose of 1 mg/kg to 1.2 mg/kg.

To successfully perform RSI, IV medications are given in rapid succession without attempts to mask ventilate to theoretically reduce the risk of aspiration. The application of cricoid pressure is included in the technique to theoretically occlude the esophagus and reduce the risk of gastric aspiration during the intubation. Cricoid pressure should be applied during the induction process and not released until correct endotracheal placement is confirmed. Confirmation is made using multiple signs: visualization of equal chest rise, positive auscultation of bilateral breath sounds, and the chemical confirmation of positive end-tidal CO_2. Anesthesia can be maintained with an inhalational volatile gas or with propofol infusion.

Propofol for very small pediatric patients

Many experienced pediatric practitioners routinely intubate infants and toddler-aged children to avoid airway problems. Infant, neonate, and premature infants are considered separate categories of patients with increased anesthetic risks.[10] The decision to intubate very small pediatric patients should be weighed against issues that may occur with instrumenting the airway, potentially causing inflammation or trauma and possibly increasing the incidence of postoperative airway complications. There is no consensus among pediatric anesthesia providers concerning an age cutoff to routinely intubate patients.

In any case, the routine intubation of all children undergoing upper GI procedures is not supported in the anesthesia literature.[27] Furthermore, there is no evidence to support the practice of routinely intubating patients who have ruled in for anesthesia care based on exclusion criteria or who have failed IV sedations.

Nonanesthesiologist-administered propofol for children

Given its high potential to induce respiratory depression and cardiovascular instability, propofol has been routinely administered by anesthesiologists for pediatric endoscopy.[64] Nevertheless, a growing number of pediatric gastroenterologists have discussed using propofol in their own practices, almost entirely without the assistance or supervision of an anesthesiologist.[2] Nonanesthesiologist-administered propofol sedation (NAAPS) describes the administration of propofol under the direction of a physician by an appropriately qualified registered nurse or physician who has not been trained as an anesthesiologist.[27] In NAAPS, propofol may be used either alone or in combination with 1 or more other agents, and a level of moderate-to-deep sedation is targeted. There has been little published regarding the use of NAAPS for pediatric procedures.

RESCUE STRATEGIES FOR COMPLICATIONS OF SEDATION

A fundamental skill in providing sedation is the ability to recognize and rescue patients from its complications. Reversal agents are available for benzodiazepines and narcotics and should be used in cases of oversedation due these agents. There are no reversal agents for other sedatives routinely used for pediatric endoscopy, including ketamine and propofol. **Table 2** lists reversal agents and their recommended dosages for children. Reversal effects are nearly always shorter than the effects of the sedatives being reversed. As such, most endoscopy guidelines stipulate that patients who receive a dose of a reversal agent should be monitored for an extended period and should be administered repeat doses if necessary.

Regardless of type of sedation used, or anesthesiologist presence, airway rescue tools should be immediately and easily accessible in all GI procedure rooms. In particular, all sizes of LMAs and endotracheal tubes; bag valve masks for delivering positive pressure ventilation; laryngoscopes, nasopharyngeal, and oropharyngeal tubes; and dedicated suction by a patient's head should be stocked. In an emer gency, the gastroenterologist should be trained and able to insert an LMA if needed.[3]

FUTURE DIRECTIONS OF SEDATION FOR PEDIATRIC ENDOSCOPY

As with all providers, pediatric gastroenterologists must continue to seek safe, efficient, and cost-effective means of providing sedation critical to performing procedures in children, which carry their own unique considerations and risks. Over time, it is possible that pediatric endoscopists will ultimately add NAAPS to the variety of options available. There has also been growing interest in developing sophisticated IV delivery systems capable of integrating patient data into computerized programs to guide drug delivery. Currently, this strategy is used to explore a safe delivery system for NAAPS that is denoted as computer-assisted personalized sedation (CAPS).

The goal of CAPS is to provide moderate sedation with propofol, with patients still able to respond to verbal or tactile instructions. Initial outcomes data suggest it is well received by adult patients and endoscopists. Postprocedure assessments by anesthesiologists also correlate well with clinically significant decisions made by the CAPS device, suggesting the software may be promising.[65]

In conclusion, sedation for pediatric endoscopy is a fundamental component of the procedure. Although patient safety must be ensured, it is also becoming increasingly important to consider efficiency and costs when choosing the type of sedation for a patient's procedure. Over the past decade, it has become standard in many pediatric gastroenterology practices to perform procedures with anesthesiologist-administered sedation, often propofol based. This evolution in practice, however, should not excuse pediatric endoscopists from remaining comfortable with common sedation regimens or from engaging in a dialogue with their anesthesiology colleagues. At the same time, anesthesiologists providing sedation for pediatric endoscopy must become knowledgeable about the various procedures for which they are sedating children and avoid unwarranted variations in care that detract from their quality. Both pediatric endoscopists and all providers involved with sedation for pediatric GI procedures should know the benefits and risks associated with various sedation regimens if they are to best advocate for their patients and their practice.

REFERENCES

1. Lightdale JR, Mahoney LB, Schwarz SM, et al. Methods of sedation in pediatric endoscopy: a survey of NASPGHAN members. J Pediatr Gastroenterol Nutr 2007;45:500–2.
2. van Beek EJ, Leroy PL. Safe and effective procedural sedation for gastrointestinal endoscopy in children. J Pediatr Gastroenterol Nutr 2012;54:171–85.
3. Vargo JJ, DeLegge MH, Feld AD, et al. Multisociety sedation curriculum for gastrointestinal endoscopy. Gastrointest Endosc 2012;76:e1–25.
4. Sheahan CG, Mathews DM. Monitoring and delivery of sedation. Br J Anaesth 2014;113(Suppl 2):ii37–47.
5. Lightdale JR, Valim C, Mahoney LB, et al. Agitation during procedural sedation and analgesia in children. Clin Pediatr (Phila) 2010;49:35–42.
6. Lightdale JR, Acosta R, Shergill AK, et al. Modifications in endoscopic practice for pediatric patients. Gastrointest Endosc 2014;79:699–710.

7. Lightdale JR, Valim C, Newburg AR, et al. Efficiency of propofol versus midazolam and fentanyl sedation at a pediatric teaching hospital: a prospective study. Gastrointest Endosc 2008;67:1067–75.

8. Miqdady MI, Hayajneh WA, Abdelhadi R, et al. Ketamine and midazolam sedation for pediatric gastrointestinal endoscopy in the Arab world. World J Gastroenterol 2011;17:3630–5.

9. Orel R, Brecelj J, Dias JA, et al. Review on sedation for gastrointestinal tract endoscopy in children by non-anesthesiologists. World J Gastrointest Endosc 2015;7:895–911.

10. Biber JL, Allareddy V, Allareddy V, et al. Prevalence and predictors of adverse events during procedural sedation anesthesia-outside the operating room for esophagogastroduodenoscopy and colonoscopy in children: age is an independent predictor of outcomes. Pediatr Crit Care Med 2015;16:e251–9.

11. Ament ME, Christie DL. Upper gastrointestinal fiberoptic endoscopy in pediatric patients. Gastroenterology 1977;72:1244–8.

12. Gilger MA, Jeiven SD, Barrish JO, et al. Oxygen desaturation and cardiac arrhythmias in children during esophagogastroduodenoscopy using conscious sedation. Gastrointest Endosc 1993;39:392–5.

13. Thakkar K, El-Serag HB, Mattek N, et al. Complications of pediatric EGD: a 4-year experience in PEDS-CORI. Gastrointest Endosc 2007;65:213–21.

14. Mamula P, Markowitz JE, Neiswender K, et al. Safety of intravenous midazolam and fentanyl for pediatric GI endoscopy: prospective study of 1578 endoscopies. Gastrointest Endosc 2007;65:203–10.

15. Lightdale JR. Sedation for pediatric endoscopy. Tech Gastrointest Endosc 2012; 15:3–8.

16. Rex DK, Overley C, Kinser K, et al. Safety of propofol administered by registered nurses with gastroenterologist supervision in 2000 endoscopic cases. Am J Gastroenterol 2002;97:1159–63.

17. Walker JA, McIntyre RD, Schleinitz PF, et al. Nurse-administered propofol sedation without anesthesia specialists in 9152 endoscopic cases in an ambulatory surgery center. Am J Gastroenterol 2003;98:1744–50.

18. Rex DK, Overley CA, Walker J. Registered nurse-administered propofol sedation for upper endoscopy and colonoscopy: Why? When? How? Rev Gastroenterol Disord 2003;3:70–80.

19. Rex DK, Heuss LT, Walker JA, et al. Trained registered nurses/endoscopy teams can administer propofol safely for endoscopy. Gastroenterology 2005;129:1384–91.

20. Lightdale JR, Mitchell PD, Fredette ME, et al. A pilot study of Ketamine versus midazolam/fentanyl sedation in children undergoing GI endoscopy. Int J Pediatr 2011;2011:623710.

21. American Society of Anesthesiology. Continuum of depth of sedation. 2011. Available at: http://www.asahq.org/for-members/. Accessed January 16, 2016.

22. Fox V. Upper gastrointestinal endoscopy. In: Walker WA, Durie PR, Hamilton JR, et al, editors. Pediatric gastrointestinal disease: pathophysiology, diagnosis, management. St Louis (MO): Mosby; 2000. p. 1514–32.

23. Liacouras CA, Mascarenhas M, Poon C, et al. Placebo-controlled trial assessing the use of oral midazolam as a premedication to conscious sedation for pediatric endoscopy. Gastrointest Endosc 1998;47:455–60.

24. Distinguishing monitored anesthesia care ("MAC" from moderate sedation/analgesia (conscious sedation). (Approved by the ASA house of delegates on October 27, 2004). 2004. Available at: http://www.asahq.org/publicationsAndServices/standards/35.pdf. Accessed January 17, 2016.

25. Mahoney LB, Lightdale JR. Sedation of the pediatric and adolescent patient for GI procedures. Curr Treat Options Gastroenterol 2007;10:412–21.
26. Dial S, Silver P, Bock K, et al. Pediatric sedation for procedures titrated to a desired degree of immobility results in unpredictable depth of sedation. Pediatr Emerg Care 2001;17:414–20.
27. Rajasekaran S, Hackbarth RM, Davis AT, et al. The safety of propofol sedation for elective nonintubated esophagogastroduodenoscopy in pediatric patients. Pediatr Crit Care Med 2014;15:e261–9.
28. Friedlander JA, DeBoer EM, Soden JS, et al. Unsedated transnasal esophago-scopy for monitoring therapy in pediatric eosinophilic esophagitis. Gastrointest Endosc 2016;83:299–306.e1.
29. Bishop PR, Nowicki MJ, May WL, et al. Unsedated upper endoscopy in children. Gastrointest Endosc 2002;55:624–30.
30. Kupietzky A. Treating very young patients with conscious sedation and medical immobilization: a Jewish perspective. Alpha Omegan 2005;98:33–7.
31. Shafran Y, Kupietzky A. General anesthesia of conscious sedation with restraint: treating the young child from a Jewish ethical perspective. J Jew Med Ethics Halacha 2005;V:29–39.
32. Walco GA, Cassidy RC, Schechter NL. Pain, hurt, and harm. The ethics of pain control in infants and children. N Engl J Med 1994;331:541–4.
33. Practice guidelines for sedation and analgesia by non-anesthesiologists. A report by the American society of anesthesiologists task force on sedation and analgesia by non-anesthesiologists. Anesthesiology 1996;84:459–71.
34. Gilger MA. Conscious sedation for endoscopy in the pediatric patient. Gastroenterol Nurs 1993;16:75–9 [discussion: 80].
35. Squires RH Jr, Morriss F, Schluterman S, et al. Efficacy, safety, and cost of intra-venous sedation versus general anesthesia in children undergoing endoscopic procedures. Gastrointest Endosc 1995;41:99–104.
36. Lewis Claar R, Walker LS, Barnard JA. Children's knowledge, anticipatory anxiety, procedural distress, and recall of esophagogastroduodenoscopy. J Pediatr Gastroenterol Nutr 2002;34:68–72.
37. Beach ML, Cohen DM, Gallagher SM, et al. Major adverse events and relation-ship to nil per Os status in pediatric sedation/anesthesia outside the operating room: a report of the pediatric sedation research consortium. Anesthesiology 2016;124:80–8.
38. Lopez-Gil M, Brimacombe J, Diaz-Reganon G. Anesthesia for pediatric gastros-copy: a study comparing the ProSeal laryngeal mask airway with nasal cannulae. Paediatr Anaesth 2006;16:1032–5.
39. Vargo JJ, Zuccaro G Jr, Dumot JA, et al. Automated graphic assessment of res-piratory activity is superior to pulse oximetry and visual assessment for the detec-tion of early respiratory depression during therapeutic upper endoscopy. Gastrointest Endosc 2002;55:826–31.
40. Colman Y, Krauss B. Microstream capnograpy technology: a new approach to an old problem. J Clin Monit Comput 1999;15:403–9.
41. Lightdale JR, Goldmann DA, Feldman HA, et al. Microstream Capnography Improves Patient Monitoring During Moderate Sedation: A Randomized, Controlled Trial. Pediatrics 2006;117:1170–8.
42. Tolia V, Peters JM, Gilger MA. Sedation for pediatric endoscopic procedures. J Pediatr Gastroenterol Nutr 2000;30:477–85.
43. Arandia HY, Patil VU. Glottic closure following large doses of fentanyl. Anesthesi-ology 1987;66:574–5.

44. Balsells F, Wyllie R, Kay M, et al. Use of conscious sedation for lower and upper gastrointestinal endoscopic examinations in children, adolescents, and young adults: a twelve-year review. Gastrointest Endosc 1997;45:375–80.

45. Koehntop DE, Rodman JH, Brundage DM, et al. Pharmacokinetics of fentanyl in neonates. Anesth Analg 1986;65:227–32.

46. Tolia V, Brennan S, Aravind MK, et al. Pharmacokinetic and pharmacodynamic study of midazolam in children during esophagogastroduodenoscopy. J Pediatr 1991;119:467–71.

47. Salonen M, Kanto J, Iisalo E, et al. Midazolam as an induction agent in children: a pharmacokinetic and clinical study. Anesth Analg 1987;66:625–8.

48. Jacobsen J, Flachs H, Dich-Nielsen JO, et al. Comparative plasma concentration profiles after i.v., i.m. and rectal administration of pethidine in children. Br J Anaesth 1988;60:623–6.

49. Gremse DA, Kumar S, Sacks AI. Conscious sedation with high-dose midazolam for pediatric gastrointestinal endoscopy. South Med J 1997;90:821–5.

50. Green SM, Nakamura R, Johnson NE. Ketamine sedation for pediatric procedures: Part 1, a prospective series. Ann Emerg Med 1990;19:1024–32.

51. Motamed F, Aminpour Y, Hashemian H, et al. Midazolam-ketamine combination for moderate sedation in upper GI endoscopy. J Pediatr Gastroenterol Nutr 2012;54:422–6.

52. Gilger MA, Spearman RS, Dietrich CL, et al. Safety and effectiveness of ketamine as a sedative agent for pediatric GI endoscopy. Gastrointestinal endoscopy 2004;59:659–63.

53. Aggarwal A, Ganguly S, Anand VK, et al. Efficacy and safety of intravenous ketamine for sedation and analgesia during pediatric endoscopic procedures. Indian Pediatr 1998;35:1211–4.

54. Green SM, Klooster M, Harris T, et al. Ketamine sedation for pediatric gastroenterology procedures. J Pediatr Gastroenterol Nutr 2001;32:26–33.

55. Khoshoo V, Thoppil D, Landry L, et al. Propofol versus midazolam plus meperidine for sedation during ambulatory esophagogastroduodenoscopy. J Pediatr Gastroenterol Nutr 2003;37:146–9.

56. Kaddu R, Bhattacharya D, Metriyakool K, et al. Propofol compared with general anesthesia for pediatric GI endoscopy: is propofol better? Gastrointest Endosc 2002;55:27–32.

57. Disma N, Astuto M, Rizzo G, et al. Propofol sedation with fentanyl or midazolam during oesophagogastroduodenoscopy in children. Eur J Anaesthesiol 2005;22:848–52.

58. Elitsur Y, Blankenship P, Lawrence Z. Propofol sedation for endoscopic procedures in children. Endoscopy 2000;32:788–91.

59. Schuttler J, Ihmsen H. Population pharmacokinetics of propofol: a multicenter study. Anesthesiology 2000;92:727–38.

60. Eyres R. Update on TIVA. Paediatr Anaesth 2004;14:374–9.

61. Cohen S, Glatstein MM, Scolnik D, et al. Propofol for pediatric colonoscopy: the experience of a large, tertiary care pediatric hospital. Am J Ther 2014;21:509–11.

62. VanNatta ME, Rex DK. Propofol alone titrated to deep sedation versus propofol in combination with opioids and/or benzodiazepines and titrated to moderate sedation for colonoscopy. Am J Gastroenterol 2006;101:2209–17.

63. Engelhardt T, Weiss M. A child with a difficult airway: what do I do next? Curr Opin Anaesthesiol 2012;25:326–32.

64. Koh JL, Black DD, Leatherman IK, et al. Experience with an anesthesiologist interventional model for endoscopy in a pediatric hospital. J Pediatr Gastroenterol Nutr 2001;33:314–8.
65. Pambianco DJ, Whitten CJ, Moerman A, et al. An assessment of computer-assisted personalized sedation: a sedation delivery system to administer propofol for gastrointestinal endoscopy. Gastrointest Endosc 2008;68:542–7.

Sedation Challenges
Obesity and Sleep Apnea

Pichamol Jirapinyo, MD[a,b], Christopher C. Thompson, MD, MSc[a,b],*

KEYWORDS

- Bariatric endoscopy • Sedation • Obesity • Anesthesia • Endoscopy
- Colonoscopy • Gastric bypass

KEY POINTS

- There is little evidence regarding endoscopic sedation in obesity and obstructive sleep apnea.
- Moderate sedation is likely safe for diagnostic and simple therapeutic procedures in the general obese and bariatric populations.
- Anesthesia support should be considered for more complicated therapeutic procedures and in the superobese.

Obesity has become an epidemic health problem worldwide. Defined as a body mass index (BMI) of greater than or equal to 30 kg/m^2, obesity is divided into class I (BMI 30–34.9 kg/m^2), class II or severe obesity (BMI 35–39.9 kg/m^2), and class III or morbid obesity (BMI >40 kg/m^2). Some surgical literature further breaks down class III obesity into superobese, which represents those with BMI of greater than or equal to 45 or 50 kg/m^2.[1,2] In 2014, the World Health Organization (WHO) reported that 33% of adults ages 18 years and older were overweight (BMI >25 kg/m^2), and 13% were obese (BMI >30 kg/m^2).[1] In the United States, this problem has become even more severe with more than half of adults ages 20 years and older being overweight and 34.9% being obese as of 2012.[3] To date, multiple conditions have been shown to be associated with obesity, including hypertension, hyperlipidemia, diabetes, stroke, osteoarthritis, and sleep apnea.[4,5] Additionally, multiple gastrointestinal diseases, including gallbladder disease, esophageal cancer, and colon cancer, have been demonstrated to be more prevalent in patients with a higher BMI.[6,7] As a result, all gastroenterologists will inevitably encounter an increase in the number of obese patients in their practice who are undergoing endoscopy.

Sedation is an integral component of every endoscopic examination. Defined as a drug-induced state in which the level of consciousness is depressed, sedation

a Division of Gastroenterology, Hepatology and Endoscopy, Brigham and Women's Hospital, 75 Francis Street, Boston, MA 02115, USA; b Harvard Medical School, 25 Shattuck Street, Boston, MA 02115, USA
* Corresponding author. Division of Gastroenterology, Hepatology and Endoscopy, Brigham and Women's Hospital, 75 Francis Street, Boston, MA 02115, USA.
E-mail address: ccthompson@partners.org

Gastrointest Endoscopy Clin N Am 26 (2016) 527–537
http://dx.doi.org/10.1016/j.giec.2016.03.001
1052-5157/16/$ – see front matter © 2016 Elsevier Inc. All rights reserved.

provides a relief in patients' discomfort and anxiety, and allows proceduralists to focus on the endoscopic work.[8,9] Four stages of sedation have been described: minimal, moderate, deep, and general anesthesia (**Table 1**). Generally, most diagnostic and uncomplicated therapeutic upper endoscopy and colonoscopy can be successfully performed under moderate sedation, formerly known as conscious sedation. During moderate sedation, patients respond purposefully to verbal commands or tactile stimulation. For longer and more complex procedures, however, deeper levels of sedation may be required. These include deep sedation in which patients cannot be easily aroused but may respond purposefully to painful or repeated simulation and general anesthesia in which patients are unarousable to painful stimuli. To appropriately choose the level of sedation for each procedure, multiple factors need to be taken into an account. These include patient's age, comorbidities, concurrent medications, pain tolerance, and the type of endoscopic procedure being performed. This article explores the medical literature on the effect of obesity and obstructive sleep apnea (OSA) on endoscopic sedation.

OBESITY AND SEDATION

Traditionally, a higher BMI was thought to be associated with an increased risk during procedural sedation. This may be due to sleep apnea, pulmonary hypertension, and restrictive lung disease, which are more common in patients with obesity. Additionally, airway management in obese patients may prove to be more difficult due to rapid oxygen desaturation, challenges with mask ventilation and intubation, and increased susceptibility to the respiratory depressant effects of sedatives.[10] As a result, many institutions require an anesthesia consultation on all patients with a BMI of 40 and higher before any endoscopic procedures to plan out the safest and most efficacious method of sedation.

Nonbariatric Obese Population

Although anecdotally obese patients are believed to be at higher risk for procedural sedation, this perception is not extensively backed up by the medical literature. In fact, the concept of BMI being a risk factor for sedation-related adverse events (SRAEs) has only recently gained an interest among gastroenterologists. In large national studies using the Clinical Outcomes Research Initiative National Endoscopic

Table 1 Four stages of sedation				
	Responsiveness	**Airway**	**Spontaneous Ventilation**	**Cardiovascular Function**
Minimal sedation	Normal response to verbal stimulation	Unaffected	Unaffected	Unaffected
Moderate sedation	Purposeful response to verbal or tactile stimulation	No intervention required	Adequate	Usually maintained
Deep sedation	Purposeful response after repeated or painful stimulation	Intervention may be required	May be inadequate	Usually maintained
General anesthesia	Unarousable even with painful stimuli	Intervention often required	Frequently inadequate	May be impaired

Data from Gross JB, Bailey PL, Connis RT, et al. Practice guidelines for sedation and analgesia by nonanesthesiologists. Anesthesiology 2002;96:1004–17.

Database (CORI-NED) in 2004 and 2007, BMI was not included in the analyses as a potential risk factor for cardiopulmonary unplanned events during endoscopy.[11,12] In these studies, patient's age, male gender, higher American Society of Anesthesiologists (ASA) classification grade, inpatient status, trainee participation, and routine use of oxygen were associated with a higher incidence of cardiopulmonary unplanned events.

Available data on the use of sedation in obese patients remained quite sparse. Most were small case series and mainly evaluated the obese patients who were undergoing advanced endoscopic procedures or upper endoscopy before a bariatric surgery. Dhariwal and colleagues[13] demonstrated in a case series of 82 subjects undergoing diagnostic upper endoscopy that a BMI greater than 28 was a risk factor for hypoxemia. In this study, other risk factors included age greater than 65 years and anemia with a hemoglobin less than 10 g/dL. Similarly, Qadeer and colleagues[14] found that a higher BMI was an independent risk factor for hypoxemia in subjects with ASA classes I and II. In this study, 79 subjects undergoing outpatient upper endoscopy, colonoscopy, endoscopic retrograde cholangiopancreatography (ERCP), and endoscopic ultrasonography (EUS) were included. Other risk factors in this study were age older than 60 years and the total dose of narcotics. Subsequently, Berzin and colleagues[15] conducted a study to assess risk factors of SRAEs during ERCP. The study included 528 subjects undergoing ERCP under deep sedation and general anesthesia. Higher ASA class and BMI higher than 30 were found to be associated with increased risk of cardiopulmonary unplanned events during ERCP. Last but not least, to better understand the optimal method of sedation for patients with a higher BMI, Mahan and colleagues[16] performed a randomized trial of 100 morbidly obese subjects (BMI≥40) who underwent upper endoscopy before bariatric surgery. In this study, the subjects were randomized to endoscopist-administered sedation with benzodiazepines and narcotics versus anesthesiologist-administered sedation with propofol. The study showed that significantly fewer patients in the anesthesiologist-administered sedation group remembered gagging during the procedure and/or complained of throat pain after the procedure. Therefore, it was concluded that deep sedation should be considered in patients undergoing preoperative upper endoscopy before bariatric surgery. Of note, in this study, hypoxemia and other cardiopulmonary unplanned events were not assessed, potentially because of the small sample size. Therefore, no conclusions regarding procedural safety can be derived from this study. Of note, to date, there have been no studies that specifically assess the safety of performing endoscopy under moderate sedation in the superobese population.

Both anatomic and metabolic factors likely play a role in sedation challenges in the obese population. An altered airway anatomy found in obese patients has been shown to be associated with difficult endotracheal intubation. In 1985, Mallampati and colleagues[17] developed and validated the Mallampati score to predict the ease of endotracheal intubation. The test consisted of a visual assessment of the distance from the tongue base to the roof of the mouth (**Figs. 1** and **2, Tables 2** and **3**).[18] A higher Mallampati score (class 3 or 4) has been shown to be associated with more difficult intubation. Subsequently, anesthesia literature has demonstrated an association between a higher Mallampati score and a higher BMI to a higher risk of intubation.[19,20] However, to date, there have been no studies that specifically demonstrate that an advanced Mallampati score leads to increased risk of sedation during endoscopy. In addition to anatomic factors, obese patients seem to metabolize sedative agents differently compared with lean patients. Specifically, binding and elimination of drugs and volumes of distribution seem more unpredictable in obese patients. Higher BMI is also likely associated with higher adipose mass, a reduction in total

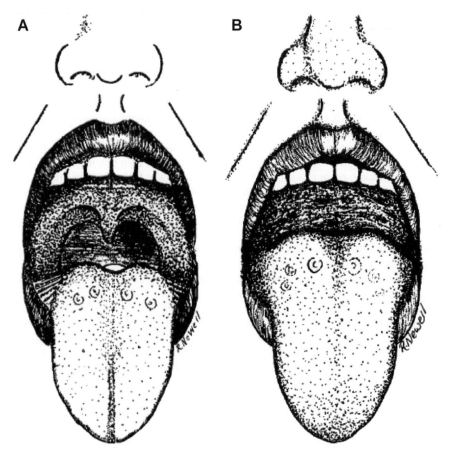

Fig. 1. Original Mallampati score. (*A*) Mallampati class 1. Faucial pillars, soft palate, and uvula are visible. (*B*) Mallampati class 3. Only soft palate is visible. (*Data from* Mallampati S, Gatt SP, Gugino LD, et al. A clinical sign to predict difficult tracheal intubation: a prospective study. Can Anaesth Soc J 1985;32:488.)

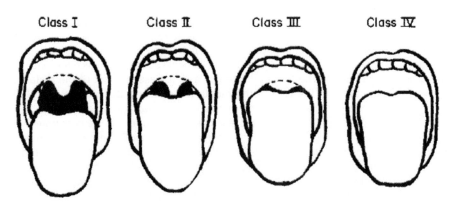

Fig. 2. Modified Mallampati score. (*Data from* Samsoon GL, Young JR. Difficult tracheal intubation. Anaesthesia 1987;42:488; with permission.)

Table 2 Original Mallampati score	
Class 1	Faucial pillars, soft palate, and uvula could be visualized
Class 2	Faucial pillars and soft palate could be visualized but uvula was masked by the base of the tongue
Class 3	Only soft palate could be visualized

Data from Mallampati S, Gatt SP, Gugino LD, et al. A clinical sign to predict difficult tracheal intubation: a prospective study. Can Anaesth Soc J 1985;32:429–34.

body water, higher glomerular filtration rate and normal hepatic clearance, which may lead to higher sedative dose requirement and thus increased sedation risks.[21]

Given the sparse literature on a direct association between a higher BMI and increased SRAEs, most society guidelines on sedation in obesity are based on expert opinion. The ASA Task Force on Sedation and Analgesia by Nonanesthesiologists mentioned that some pre-existing comorbidities may be related to adverse outcomes in patients receiving either moderate or deep sedation. These risk factors include significant obesity, especially if it involves the neck and facial structures.[22] Similarly, the American Gastroenterological Association Institute review of endoscopic sedation recommended the use of an anesthesia professional for patients who are morbidly obese (BMI≥40).[13] However, this is an expert opinion only and no supportive evidence was provided.[23]

Bariatric Population

With the worsening obesity epidemic, the number of bariatric surgeries being performed has also increased. In 2013, about 179,000 bariatric surgeries were performed in the United States. Of these, more than one-third were Roux-en-Y gastric bypass (RYGB).[24] Although RYGB results in relatively durable weight loss and an improvement in presurgical comorbidities, postoperative complications, including anastomotic leak, gastrogastric fistula, marginal ulceration, and weight regain, are not uncommon.[25,26] To manage these complications effectively, an endoscopic examination is usually required.

Anecdotally, bariatric patients have been observed to require higher sedative doses than those without a history of bariatric surgery, which leads to increased sedation risks. Some institutions require an anesthesia professional during any endoscopic examination performed on RYGB patients, which usually leads to longer wait time and greater economic burden. Similar to nonbariatric obese patients, data on the use of sedation in the bariatric population remain very sparse. Jirapinyo and colleagues[27] reported that it was safe to perform upper endoscopy in the RYGB using moderate sedation, without anesthesia support. In this study, unplanned events were reported to be 1.6%, with 0.6% being cardiopulmonary unplanned events. This was

Table 3 Modified Mallampati score	
Class I	Soft palate, uvula, fauces, pillars visible
Class II	Soft palate, uvula, fauces visible
Class III	Soft palate, base of uvula visible
Class IV	Only hard palate visible

Data from Samsoon GL, Young JR. Difficult tracheal intubation. Anaesthesia 1987;42:487–90.

relatively similar to the reported SRAEs in the general population, which varied from 0.13% in Silvis and colleagues[28] to 0.9% in Sharma and colleagues.[11] In this study, procedural length, and not absolute BMI, was the predictor of sedation requirement in the RYGB population. A subsequent matched cohort study from the same group showed that RYGB subjects required higher doses of sedation during esophagogastroduodenoscopy (EGD) than the non-RYGB with similar age, gender, and BMI.[29] The investigators hypothesized that these findings could be due to an improvement in liver function after gastric bypass, which resulted in an improvement in liver metabolism of fentanyl and midazolam, which subsequently led to increased requirement of both sedatives during EGD.[30,31]

Based on the currently limited available data, performing uncomplicated upper endoscopy in the RYGB seems to be safe and effective under endoscopist-directed moderate sedation. However, more studies are needed regarding sedation choice for colonoscopy and other endoscopic procedures.

OBSTRUCTIVE SLEEP APNEA AND SEDATION

OSA is a sleep disorder that is defined as repetitive total or partial collapses of the upper airway causing episodes of apnea and hypopnea during sleep. It is found in about 4% of men and 2% of women.[32] Although being overweight or obese is a strong risk factor, OSA may also occur in the nonobese population with the following risk factors: male gender, age older than 40, neck size larger than 16 or 17 inches, enlarged tonsils, enlarged tongue, gastroesophageal reflux disease, family history of sleep apnea, and smoking.[33] The diagnosis of OSA requires clinical symptoms and the results of a formal sleep study (polysomnography). The Apnea Hypopnea Index (AHI) is an index used to indicate the severity of OSA. It is defined as the number of apneas or hypopneas recorded during the study per hour of sleep. Mild OSA has 5 to 14.9 events per hour of sleep, moderate OSA falls in the range of 15 to 29.9 events per hour of sleep, and severe OSA has more than 30 events per hour of sleep.

It is thought that the presence of OSA may increase the risk of cardiopulmonary unplanned events during endoscopy. Anecdotally, some endoscopy units have required patients with known OSA bring their continuous positive airway ventilation (CPAP) for use during procedure recovery. However, similar to data on sedation in obesity, medical literature to support this concept remains somewhat conflicting. Khaini and colleagues[34] studied the incidence of hypoxemia (pulse oximetry <92%) in 233 subjects undergoing elective outpatient upper endoscopy and colonoscopy under moderate sedation using a combination of benzodiazepine and an opioid. In this study, the subjects were divided into high-risk (39%) and low-risk (61%) for OSA using the Berlin Questionnaire, which assessed snoring, daytime somnolence, and hypertension and BMI (**Box 1**) in subjects with no known formal diagnosis of OSA.[35] There was no significant difference in the incidence of hypoxemia between the high-risk and low-risk groups (odds ratio 1.48, 95% CI 0.58–3.80).[34] The investigators suggested that this finding might be due to the subject cohort being relatively healthy. As a result, in the setting of relatively brief procedures targeting moderate sedation, there seemed to be no added risk in subjects thought to be at risk for OSA. For patients requiring deeper sedation, however, data in the literature remains more varied. Cote and colleagues assessed the sedation risk in 231 subjects undergoing advanced procedures, including EUS and ERCP under deep sedation or general anesthesia. The STOP-BANG (SB) Questionnaire was used to screen subjects with undiagnosed OSA in the preprocedural setting (**Table 4**). It provides a quick, reproducible score

Box 1
Berlin Questionnaire

Category 1: Snoring

1. Do you snore?
   a. Yes
   b. No
   c. Do not know

2. Your snoring is
   a. Slightly louder than breathing
   b. As loud as talking
   c. Louder than talking

3. How often do you snore?
   a. Almost every day
   b. 3 to 4 times per week
   c. 1 to 2 times per week
   d. 1 to 2 times per month
   e. Rarely or never

4. Has your snoring ever bothered other people?
   a. Yes
   b. No
   c. Do not know

5. Has anyone noticed that you stop breathing during your sleep?
   a. Almost every day
   b. 3 to 4 times per week
   c. 1 to 2 times per week
   d. 1 to 2 times per month
   e. Rarely or never

Category 2: Daytime somnolence

6. How often do you feel tired or fatigued after you sleep?
   a. Almost every day
   b. 3 to 4 times per week
   c. 1 to 2 times per week
   d. 1 to 2 times per month
   e. Rarely or never

7. During your waking time, do you feel tired, fatigued, or not up to par?
   a. Almost every day
   b. 3 to 4 times per week
   c. 1 to 2 times per week
   d. 1 to 2 times per month
   e. Rarely or never

8. Have you ever nodded off or fallen asleep while driving a vehicle?
   a. Yes
   b. No

9. How often does this occur?
   a. Almost every day
   b. 3 to 4 times per week
   c. 1 to 2 times per week
   d. 1 to 2 times per month
   e. Rarely or never

Category 3: Hypertension and BMI

10. Do you have high blood pressure?
    a. Yes
    b. No
    c. Do not know

BMI = ?

Category 1. Item 1: if Yes, assign 1 point; item 2: if c or d is the response, assign 1 point; item 3: if a or b is the response, assign 1 point; item 4: if a is the response, assign 1 point; item 5: if a or b is the response, assign 2 points Add points. Category 1 is positive if the total score is 2 or more points.

Category 2. Items 6, 7, 8 (item 9 should be noted separately). Item 6: if a or b is the response, assign 1 point; item 7: if a or b is the response, assign 1 point; item 8: if a is the response, assign 1 point. Add points. Category 2 is positive if the total score is 2 or more points.

Category 3 is positive if the answer to item 10 is Yes or if the BMI of the patient is greater than 30 kg/m^2.

High-risk: if there are 2 or more categories for which the score is positive.

Low-risk: if there are only 1 or no categories for which the score is positive.

Data from Netzer NC, Stoohs RA, Netzer CM, et al. Using the Berlin Questionnaire to identify patients at risk for the sleep apnea syndrome. Ann Intern Med 1999;131:485–91.

from 8 yes or no questions (1 point each) that predicts patients with moderate to severe OSA. Of note, a prospective validation study demonstrated that a positive SB (score$\geq$3) has a sensitivity of 83.6% and 92.9% in predicting an AHI score of greater than 5 (mild sleep apnea) and an AHI of greater than or equal to 15 (moderate to severe sleep apnea).[36] Cote and colleagues[37] showed that subjects with a positive SB score had a higher incidence of hypoxemia and the need for airway maneuvers such as a chin lift or placement of a nasopharyngeal airway. In contradistinction, Mehta and colleagues[38] reported that a higher SB score was not associated with an increased incidence of SRAEs or with airway intervention in their study cohort of 243 subjects undergoing upper endoscopy or colonoscopy under anesthesiologist-directed propofol sedation. A higher BMI, however, was associated with an increased incidence of both outcomes.

Given the currently available data, the ASA guideline recommends that capnography or other automated devices should be used for monitoring of ventilation in patients with OSA who are undergoing procedures under moderate sedation.[8,39] CPAP monitoring may also be considered in this setting. Similarly, the American Society for Gastrointestinal Endoscopy guidelines suggest that a history of sleep apnea, snoring, and stridor should be reviewed as part of the pre-endoscopic assessment because patients with OSA may be at increased risk for sedation-related complications during endoscopic examination.[40]

Table 4
STOP-BANG Questionnaire

S	Snoring: Do you snore loudly (louder than talking or loud enough to be heard through closed doors)?	Yes/No
T	Tired: Do you often feel tired, fatigued, or sleepy during the daytime?	Yes/No
O	Observed: Has anyone observed you stop breathing during your sleep?	Yes/No
P	Blood pressure: Have you or are you being treated for high blood pressure?	Yes/No
B	BMI: >35 kg/m^2	Yes/No
A	Age: Age older than 50 y	Yes/No
N	Neck circumference: >40 cm	Yes/No
G	Gender: Male	Yes/No

High risk of OSA: yes to 3 or more questions; low risk of OSA: yes to less than 3 questions.

Data from Chung F, Yegneswaran B, Liao P, et al. STOP questionnaire: a tool to screen patients for obstructive sleep apnea. Anesthesiology 2008;108:812–21.

SUMMARY

Data on endoscopic sedation in patients with obesity and OSA remain quite sparse. Most society guidelines on sedation in this patient population are based on expert opinions only. Most studies seem to suggest increased sedation requirement and risk of adverse events in patients with obesity and OSA. However, to date, there has been no objective way to quantify this risk pre-endoscopically to designate the appropriate level of sedation and personnel before the procedure. In general, for most diagnostic and uncomplicated therapeutic upper endoscopy, data seem to demonstrate that it is safe and effective to perform the procedure under moderate sedation with a combination of benzodiazepine and opioids. For a longer and more complex procedure or for superobese patients, however, it seems prudent to arrange for anesthesia support. Until more population-based studies or randomized studies are available, performing endoscopy in this patient population should always alert providers to plan carefully and individualize sedation plans for every patient.

REFERENCES

1. WHO. Global status report on noncommunicable diseases 2014. Geneva (Switzerland): World Health Organization; 2015.
2. Sturm R. Increase in morbid obesity in the USA: 2000-2005. Public Health 2007; 121:492–6.
3. Ogden CL, Carroll MD, Kit BK, et al. Prevalence of childhood and adult obesity in the United States, 2011-2012. JAMA 2014;311:806–14.
4. Khaodhiar L, McCowen KC, Blackburn GL. Obesity and its comorbid conditions. Clin Cornerstone 1999;2:17–31.
5. Guh DP, Zhang W, Bansback N, et al. The incidence of co-morbidities related to obesity and overweight: a systematic review and meta-analysis. BMC Public Health 2009;9:88.
6. Chen Q, Zhuang H, Liu Y. The association between obesity factor and esophageal cancer. J Gastrointest Oncol 2012;3:226–31.
7. Frezza EE, Wachtel MS, Chiriva-Internati M. Influence of obesity on the risk of developing colon cancer. Gut 2006;55:285–91.
8. Gross JB, Bailey PL, Connis RT, et al. Practice guidelines for sedation and analgesia by non-anesthesiologists. Anesthesiology 2002;96:1004–17.
9. Faigel DO, Baron TH, Goldstein JL, et al. Standards practice committee, American Society for Gastrointestinal Endoscopy: guidelines for the use of deep sedation and anesthesia for GI endoscopy. Gastrointest Endosc 2002;56:613–7.
10. Schumann R. Anaesthesia for bariatric surgery. Best Pract Res Clin Anaesthesiol 2011;25:83–93.
11. Sharma VK, Nguyen CC, Crowell MD, et al. A national study of cardiopulmonary unplanned events after GI endoscopy. Gastrointest Endosc 2007;66:27–34.
12. Gangi S, Saidi F, Patel K, et al. Cardiovascular complications after GI endoscopy: occurrence and risks in a large hospital system. Gastrointest Endosc 2004;60: 679–85.
13. Dhariwal A, Plevris JN, Lo NT, et al. Age anemia and obesity-associated oxygen desaturation during upper gastrointestinal endoscopy. Gastrointest Endosc 1992;38:684–8.
14. Qadeer MA, Lopez R, Dumot JA, et al. Risk factors for hypoxemia during ambulatory gastrointestinal endoscopy in ASA I-II patients. Dig Dis Sci 2009;54: 1035–40.

15. Berzin TM, Sanaka S, Barnett SR, et al. A prospective assessment of sedation-related adverse events and patient and endoscopist satisfaction in ERCP with anesthesiologist-administered sedation. Gastrointest Endosc 2011;73:710–7.
16. Madan A, Tichansky D, Isom J, et al. Monitored anesthesia care with propofol versus surgeon-monitored sedation with benzodiazepines and narcotics for preoperative endoscopy in the morbidly obese. Obes Surg 2008;18:545–8.
17. Mallampati S, Gatt SP, Gugino LD, et al. A clinical sign to predict difficult tracheal intubation: a prospective study. Can Anaesth Soc J 1985;32:429–34.
18. Samsoon GL, Young JR. Difficult tracheal intubation. Anaesthesia 1987;42: 487–90.
19. Hekiert AM, Mick R, Mirza N. Prediction of difficult laryngoscopy: dose obesity play a role? Ann Otol Rhinol Laryngol 2007;116:799–804.
20. Juvin P, Lavaut E, Dupont H, et al. Difficult tracheal intubation is more common in obese than in lean patients. Anesth Analg 2003;97:595–600.
21. Vargo JJ. Procedural sedation and obesity: waters left uncharted. Gastrointest Endosc 2009;70:980–4.
22. Metzner J, Posner KL, Domino KB. The risk and safety of anesthesia at remote locations: the US closed claims analysis. Curr Opin Anaesthesiol 2009;22:502–8.
23. Cohen LB, DeLegge MH, Aisenberg J, et al. AGA Institute review of endoscopic sedation. Gastroenterology 2007;133:675–701.
24. Ponce J, Nguyen NT, Hutter M, et al. American Society for Metabolic and Bariatric Surgery estimation of bariatric surgery procedures in the United States, 2011-2014. Surg Obes Relat Dis 2015;11:1199–200.
25. Sjöström L, Lindroos AK, Peltonen M, et al. Lifestyle, diabetes, and cardiovascular risk factors 10 years after bariatric surgery. N Engl J Med 2004;351:2683–93.
26. Kumar N, Thompson CC. Endoscopic management of complications after gastrointestinal weight loss surgery. Clin Gastroenterol Hepatol 2013;11:343–53.
27. Jirapinyo P, Abu Dayyeh BK, Thompson CC. Conscious sedation for upper endoscopy in the gastric bypass patient: prevalence of cardiopulmonary adverse events and predictors of sedation requirement. Dig Dis Sci 2014;59(9):2173–7.
28. Silvis SE, Nebel O, Rogers G, et al. Endoscopic complications. Results of the 1974 American Society for Gastrointestinal Endoscopy Survey. JAMA 1976;235: 928–30.
29. Jirapinyo P, Kumar N, Thompson CC. Patients with roux-en-Y gastric bypass require increased sedation during upper endoscopy. Clin Gastroenterol Hepatol 2015;13(8):1432–6.
30. Tandra S, Chalasani N, Jones DR, et al. Pharmacokinetic and pharmacodynamic alterations in the Roux-en-Y gastric bypass recipients. Ann Surg 2013;258:262–9.
31. Brill MJ, van Rongen A, van Dongen EP, et al. The Pharmacokinetics of the CYP3A substrate midazolam in morbidly obese patients before and one year after bariatric surgery. Pharm Res 2015;32:3927–36.
32. Young T, Palta M, Dempsey J, et al. The occurrence of sleep disordered breathing among middle aged adults. N Engl J Med 1993;328:1230–5.
33. Young T, Skatrud J, Peppard PE. Risk factors for obstructive sleep apnea in adults. JAMA 2004;291:2013–6.
34. Khiani VS, Salah W, Maimone S, et al. Sedation during endoscopy for patients at risk for sleep apnea. Gastrointest Endosc 2009;70:1116–20.
35. Netzer NC, Stoohs RA, Netzer CM, et al. Using the Berlin questionnaire to identify patients at risk for the sleep apnea syndrome. Ann Intern Med 1999;131:485–91.
36. Chung F, Yegneswaran B, Liao P, et al. STOP questionnaire: a tool to screen patients for obstructive sleep apnea. Anesthesiology 2008;108:812–21.

37. Cote GA, Hovis CE, Hovis RM, et al. A screening instrument for sleep apnea predicts airway maneuvers in patients undergoing advanced endoscopic procedures. Clin Gastroenterol Hepatol 2010;8:660–5.
38. Mehta PP, Kochhar G, Kalra S, et al. Can a validated sleep apnea scoring system predict cardiopulmonary events using propofol sedation for routine EGD or colonoscopy? A prospective cohort study. Gastrointest Endosc 2014;79:436–44.
39. American Society of Anesthesiologists Task Force on the perioperative management of patients with obstructive sleep apnea. Practice guidelines for the perioperative management of patients with obstructive sleep apnea. Anesthesiology 2006;104: 1081–93.
40. ASGE Standards of Practice Committee. Sedation and anesthesia in GI endoscopy. Gastrointest Endosc 2008;68:205–16.

Sedation in the Ambulatory Endoscopy Center

Optimizing Safety, Expectations and Throughput

Joseph J. Vicari, MD[a,b,]*

KEYWORDS

- Optimizing safety • Patient expectations • Medication • Patient monitoring
- Efficiency

KEY POINTS

- Optimizing safety is the responsibility of the endoscopist and gastrointestinal assistant of the 21st century. Each must have expertise in sedation and analgesia and patient monitoring.
- Patient expectations must be balanced with physician expectations and safety.
- The most efficient ambulatory endoscopy center will successfully navigate changes occurring in the health care system. Safety and efficiency must be viewed as 1 process.

In the United States, sedation and analgesia are the standard of practice when endoscopic procedures are performed in the ambulatory endoscopy center (AEC). Surveys indicate that physicians and patients expect that sedation and analgesia will routinely and safely be administered for endoscopic procedures.[1,2] Over the last 30 years, there has been a dramatic shift of endoscopic procedures from the hospital outpatient department to AECs. This article will review sedation and analgesia in the AEC as it relates to optimizing safety, patient expectations, and efficiency.

OPTIMIZING SAFETY—PREPROCEDURE

The responsibilities of the endoscopist and gastrointestinal assistant of the 21st century reach beyond endoscopy. Each must have expertise in sedation and analgesia and patient monitoring, and awareness of potential complications.

a Rockford Gastroenterology Associates, Ltd, 401 Roxbury Road, Rockford, IL 61107, USA;
b Department of Medicine, University of Illinois College of Medicine at Rockford, 1601 Parkview Avenue, Rockford, IL 61107, USA
* Department of Medicine, University of Illinois College of Medicine at Rockford, 1601 Parkview Avenue, Rockford, IL 61107.
E-mail address: joevicari@msn.com

Gastrointest Endoscopy Clin N Am 26 (2016) 539–552
http://dx.doi.org/10.1016/j.giec.2016.02.005
1052-5157/16/$ – see front matter © 2016 Elsevier Inc. All rights reserved.

Sedation may be defined as a medication-induced depression in the level of consciousness.[3] The purpose of sedation and analgesia is to relieve patient anxiety and discomfort, improve the outcome of the examination, and diminish the patient's memory of the event.[3] Sedation and analgesia comprise a continuum of states ranging from minimal sedation (anxiolysis) to general anesthesia.[4]

Table 1 outlines the definitions of the levels of sedation and analgesia. Historically, in the United States, endoscopic procedures in the AEC have been performed with patients under moderate sedation using benzodiazepines and narcotics.

In the United States over the last 15 years, there has been a significant shift to deep sedation using propofol when performing endoscopic procedures in the AEC. In 2009, more than 30% of endoscopic procedures were performed under deep sedation utilizing anesthesia services.[5] In 2015, most endoscopic procedures in AECs were performed under deep sedation utilizing anesthesia services.

Preprocedure preparation and assessment include appropriate discussion of the procedure and obtaining consent. This discussion should include indications, benefits, risks, and alternatives to the procedure. There are several other important preprocedure variables to assess and implement. According to the American Society of Anesthesiologists' (ASA) practice guidelines for sedation and analgesia by nonanesthesiologists, patients should fast a minimum of 2 hours for clear liquids and 6 hours for a light meal.[4]

A history and physical examination should be performed prior to endoscopy. The examination should focus on sedation and analgesia-related issues. The following data should be collected: (1) abnormalities of major organ systems; (2) snoring, stridor, or sleep apnea; (3) drug allergies, current medications, and potential for drug interactions; (4) prior adverse reaction(s) to sedatives or anesthetics; (5) time, and type, of last oral intake; and (6) tobacco, alcohol or substance abuse.[4] The physical examination should include the following: measurement of vital signs, determination of baseline level of consciousness, and examination of the heart, lungs, and airway anatomy.[4] **Table 2** defines the ASA physical classification system.

Table 1 Levels of sedation and anesthesia				
	Minimal Sedation (Anxiolysis)	Moderate Sedation (Conscious Sedation)	Deep Sedation	General Anesthesia
Responsiveness	Normal response to verbal stimulation	Purposeful response to verbal or tactile stimulation	Purposeful response after repeated or painful stimulation	Unarousable even with painful stimulus
Airway	Unaffected	No intervention required	Intervention may be required	Intervention often required
Spontaneous ventilation	Unaffected	Adequate	May be inadequate	Frequently inadequate
Cardiovascular function	Unaffected	Usually maintained	Usually maintained	May be impaired

Modified from Gross JB, Bailey PL, Connis RT, et al. Practice guidelines for sedation and analgesia by nonanesthesiologists. Anesthesiology 2002;96:1004–17.

Table 2
ASA physical status classification system (Last approved on October 15, 2014)

ASA PS Classification	Definition	Examples, Including, but Not Limited to:
ASA I[a]	A normal healthy patient	Healthy, nonsmoking, no or minimal alcohol use
ASA II[a]	A patient with mild systemic disease	Mild diseases only without substantive functional limitations Examples include (but not limited to): current smoker, social alcohol drinker, pregnancy, obesity (30< body mass index [BMI] <40), well-controlled DM/HTN, mild lung disease
ASA III[a]	A patent with severe systemic disease	Substantive functional limitations; one or more moderate-to-severe diseases Examples include (but not limited to): poorly controlled DM or HTN, chronic obstructive pulmonary disease, morbid obesity (BMI ≥40), active hepatitis, alcohol dependence or abuse, implanted pacemaker, moderate reduction of ejection fraction, end-stage renal disease undergoing regularly scheduled dialysis, premature infant PCA <60 wk, history (>3 mo) or myocardial infarction, CVA, TIA, or CAD/stents.
ASA IV[a]	A patient with severe systemic disease that is constant threat to life	Examples include (but not limited to): recent (<3 mo) MI, CVA, TIA, or CAD/stent, ongoing cardiac ischemia or severe valve dysfunction, severe reduction of ejection fraction, sepsis, DIC, ARD, or ESRD not undergoing regularly scheduled dialysis
ASA V[a]	A moribund patient who is not expected to survive without the operation	Examples include (but not limited to): ruptured abdominal/thoracic aneurysm, massive trauma, intracranial bleed with mass effect, ischemic bowel in the face of significant cardiac pathology or multiple organ/system dysfunction
ASA VI[a]	A declared brain-dead patient whose organs are being removed for donor purposes	—

[a] The addition of "E" denotes Emergency surgery: (an emergency is defined as existing when delay in treatment of the patient would lead to a significant increase in the threat to life or body part).

Abbreviations: ARD, acute respiratory distress; CAD, coronary artery disease; CVA, cerebrovascular accident; DIC, disseminated intravascular coagulation; DM, diabetes mellitus; HTN, hypertension; PCA, patient controlled anesthesia; TIA, transient ischemic attack.

PATIENT EXPECTATIONS—SEDATION AND ANALGESIA

Historically, in the United States, moderate sedation and analgesia for endoscopic procedures were the standard of practice. Today, at least half of endoscopic procedures in the AEC are performed with monitored anesthesia care (MAC) targeting deep sedation. One of the factors leading to an increased use of MAC is patient expectation for comfort and lack of memory for the procedure. General patient expectations are similar to physician expectations: safety and comfort during endoscopy. However, many patients place more emphasis on comfort during endoscopic procedures. As patients do not fully understand the many factors involved in patient safety and performing a quality endoscopic procedure, it is important for AEC staff and endoscopists to communicate to the patient the many variables (medications, monitoring equipment, and efficiency) that affect safety, comfort, and quality in endoscopy. Safety, quality, and comfort extend beyond the actual performance of the procedure; these three factors apply to the entire experience as patients move through the AEC for the duration of their endoscopic visit.

The ideal medication for sedation and analgesia should have a rapid onset of action and produce a predictable effect. It should not precipitate cardiopulmonary decompensation. Finally, it should lead to amnesia for the period of time during which the procedure is performed and extend into the postprocedure recovery period. Ideally, the medication should be administered by the endoscopy nurse and have an acceptable safety profile. A drug such as this would meet all patient and endoscopist expectations.

MEDICATIONS

Currently, the ideal medication for sedation and analgesia for endoscopic procedures does not exist. The most common medications used for sedation and analgesia include benzodiazepines, narcotics, and propofol. Regardless of who administers the medication (nurse, endoscopist, nurse anesthetist, or anesthesiologist), the endoscopist must be familiar with all drugs given for endoscopic procedures.

Benzodiazepines

Midazolam is the most commonly used benzodiazepine for sedation and analgesia during endoscopy.[6–9] It is a sedative hypnotic that causes varying degrees of amnesia. Midazolam reaches its peak effect quickly (approximately 3–5 minutes) and has an elimination half-life of 1 to 4 hours in healthy individuals. In older patients and in those with significant comorbid disease, the half-life of may be prolonged. A typical starting dose for midazolam is 0.5 to 2 mg intravenously; subsequent dosing should be administered in 1 mg increments.

Midazolam causes antegrade amnesia. It may cause hypoventilation, which may lead to lower oxygen saturation. Hypoventilation is believed to be secondary to depression of the respiratory center in the brainstem.[9] In general, benzodiazepines have minimal effect on the cardiovascular system. With marked sedation, there is some peripheral vasodilation and a slight drop in cardiac output and peripheral resistance.[10] Subsequently, hypotension may develop.

Opioids

Fentanyl is the most commonly used opioid analgesic for sedation and analgesia during endoscopic procedures. It's typically combined with benzodiazepines. Fentanyl has a mild sedative effect and decreases the intensity of painful stimuli.[11] It reaches its peak effect in approximately 5 minutes and has a duration of action of 1 to 3 hours. A typical starting dose for fentanyl is 50 to 100 μg intravenously; subsequent dosing should be administered in 25 to 50 μg increments. The major adverse effects of fentanyl are respiratory depression with hypoxemia and CO_2 retention. Respiratory depression results from central depression of ventilatory response to CO_2 and decreased respiratory rate with or without decreased tidal volume.[11,12]

In the United States, fentanyl is not routinely used alone because of its minimal sedative effect. Opioid analgesics are generally used in combination with benzodiazepines.[2,12] Combining opioid analgesics and benzodiazepines lead to a rapid and reliable induction of sedation,[13,14] synergistic and additive effects, enhanced patient tolerance of the procedure,[7,15] and increased ability for the physician to complete the procedure.[6] Combining opioid analgesics and benzodiazepines increases the potential for an adverse event. The addition of opioid analgesics to benzodiazepines has a synergistic effect on respiratory depression and hypoxemia.[16,17] Because of these additive and synergistic effects, reduced doses should be used when combining these drugs. In general, when combining these agents, the opioid analgesic should be administered first,[17] followed by the benzodiazepines, using smaller doses of each compared with using either drug alone.[11]

Propofol

Propofol is classified as a short-acting sedative, amnestic, and hypnotic that provides minimal analgesia.[17,18] The peak effect occurs quickly, in 30 to 60 seconds, and the half-life is 1.8 to 4.1 minutes. These properties account for a quick recovery time after cessation of propofol, generally 10 to 30 minutes.[17] Propofol can be administered as a single bolus or continuous infusion and has been studied alone and in combination with benzodiazepines and opioid analgesics for endoscopy.[19–21] When propofol was combined with opioid analgesics or benzodiazepines, patients reported better tolerance of the procedure and reached a deeper level of sedation. There was no increase in adverse events when comparing the combination of propofol and fentanyl with midazolam and meperidine.[19–21] Advantages of propofol include better tolerance of endoscopy, deeper level of sedation, and more rapid recovery time.[18–20] Disadvantages of propofol include pain at the injection site, shorter amnesia span, and less analgesia.[20,22] One final disadvantage of propofol is the cost, which is higher compared with opioid analgesics and benzodiazepines. The increased cost is secondary to medication cost and the use of an anesthesia professional. **Table 3** summarizes

Table 3 Sedatives and analgesics	
Drug	**Description**
Midazolam	Sedative/hypnotic, ideal for sedation, but not analgesia. Produces amnesia when used in adequate doses (unlike diazepam and does not cause phlebitis). Respiratory depression is potentiated if given with opioids and if given by bolus rather than titrated. Peak effect: 3–5 min. Duration of action: 1–3 h. Potential side effects: respiratory depression (hypoxemia, CO_2 retention); decreased tidal volume with increased respiratory rate, apneic pauses, increased upper airway resistance. Hypotension Typical starting dose: 0.5–2 mg intravenously.
Fentanyl	Opioid analgesic with mild sedative properties: rapid onset of action and rapid recovery. Peak effect: 5–8 min. Duration of action: 1–3 h. Potential adverse effects: respiratory depression (hypoxemia and CO_2 retention); decreased respiratory rate; and possible decrease in tidal volume. Typical starting dose: 50–100 µg IU. Respiratory depression and sedation are potentiated when benzodiazepines are given concurrently with opioid narcotics.
Propofol	Short-acting sedative, amnestic, and hypnotic that provides minimal analgesia. Peak effect: 30–60 s. Half-life: 1.8–4.1 min. Potential adverse effects: pain at injection site, respiratory depression, reduction in systemic or vascular resistance with possible hypotension, and possibly pancreatitis. Typical starting dose: 25 µg/kg/min intravenous infusion, 30-min procedure may require total dose 200–400 mg.

the medication use and adverse effects. Adverse effects of propofol include respiratory depression, a reduction in systemic vascular resistance with possible hypotension, and pain on venous injection.

ANTAGONISTS

For patient safety, benzodiazepine and narcotic reversal medications are available for use in the AEC.

Antagonists

Flumazenil is a benzodiazepine antagonist that specifically blocks the central effects of benzodiazepines. The central effects of benzodiazepines are reversed 30 to 60 seconds after an intravenous injection of flumazenil.[10] The peak effect occurs in 3 to 5 minutes, and the duration of action is 1 to 2 hours. A typical starting dose of flumazenil is 0.2 mg intravenously, usually not exceeding a total dose of 1 mg. Flumazenil has been shown to shorten recovery time after sedation and potentially allow for improved efficiency in the recovery and discharge planning of patients from the endoscopy suite.[23,24] The use of reversal agents to hasten discharge has come under criticism, however, because of the problem of resedation; extended observation after reversal agents has been suggested to watch for this potential problem. Resedation may occur in patients receiving flumazenil because of its short duration of action compared with benzodiazepines. This typically occurs, however, when using larger dosages of benzodiazepines. When flumazenil was routinely used to recover patients in 2 randomized trials, resedation was not noted.[23,24] Flumazenil may provoke withdrawal seizures, particularly in patients habituated to benzodiazepines (**Table 4**).

Naloxone is an opioid antagonist used to reverse respiratory depression and central nervous system effects induced by opioid analgesics. The peak effect occurs in 1 to 2 minutes; duration of action is 1 to 3 hours. A typical starting dose of naloxone is 0.04 mg intravenously, usually not exceeding a total dose of 0.4 mg. Adverse effects include nausea, vomiting, tachycardia, arrhythmias, pulmonary edema, and sudden death in patients with cardiac disease. Because of the possible adverse effects,

Table 4 Benzodiazepine and opioid analgesic antagonists	
Drug	**Description**
Flumazenil	Reverses benzodiazepine-induced sedation. Questionable or delayed efficacy in reversing benzodiazepine-induced respiratory depression. Peak effect: 3–5 min Duration of action: 1–2 h Potential side effects: resedation, seizures (only in benzodiazepine-habituated patients) Typical starting dose: 0.2–0.5 mg intravenously, up to 1 mg
Naloxone	Reverses opioid-induced analgesia, central nervous system adverse effects and respiratory depression Peak effect: 1–2 min Duration of action: 1–3 h Potential adverse effects: pain, agitation, nausea or vomiting, tachycardia, arrhythmias, pulmonary edema, withdrawal syndrome, opioid habituated patients, renarcotization Typical starting dose: 0.04 mg intravenously for reversal of analgesia/sedation. Total dose up to 0.4 mg

routine reversal with naloxone should be avoided. Reversal of naloxone should be reserved for patients with significant respiratory depression or a respiratory arrest. As with flumazenil, naloxone can permit resedation, because its duration of action is shorter than opioid analgesics used for endoscopic procedures.

Optimizing Safety—During and After the Procedure

Patient monitoring by gastrointestinal assistants, certified registered nurse anesthetists, anesthesiologists, endoscopists, and electronic devices during sedation and analgesia for gastrointestinal endoscopy is the standard of care in the United States.

Prior to beginning an endoscopic procedure the patient, staff and endoscopist should verify the identity of the patient and procedure to be performed (time out).[25]

The primary goal of monitoring the patient is the early detection of potentially harmful changes in a patient's physiologic parameters.[1] The process of monitoring begins with the gastrointestinal assistant. A well-trained gastrointestinal assistant is necessary to assess and monitor the patient adequately during sedation and analgesia. The endoscopist cannot safely perform the procedure and adequately monitor the patient alone. If a complex or unusually long procedure is anticipated, a second gastrointestinal assistant may be necessary.

For moderate sedation and analgesia, the gastrointestinal assistant monitoring the patient may assist the endoscopist with minor interruptible tasks, as long as patient safety is not compromised. For deep sedation, a separate assistant is required to assist the endoscopist, leaving the monitoring assistant (anesthesia professional) free for continuous monitoring.

Safe medication administration practices promote safety in medication administration and have become a highly scrutinized activity within health care.[24,26,27] All medications used in gastrointestinal endoscopy should be labeled. Medications marked either on the container or noted in the package insert as single-patient use should be used for a single patient only, and any remaining drug should be discarded.[25]

Single-dose vials are preferred when administering medication to multiple patients. If a multidose vial will be used for more than 1 patient, it should remain in a centralized medication area and not enter the procedure room.[25]

Standard monitoring of the patient during moderate sedation and analgesia includes measurement of oxygen saturation, heart rate, blood pressure, and respiratory rate. Pulse oximetry provides a continuous measurement of oxygen saturation. The pulse oximeter directs an infrared beam of light into the vascular bed of the finger, then uses the optically detected color changes in the reflected light to estimate the percentage of hemoglobin bound to oxygen.[26] By detecting the color change in the reflected light, oxygen saturation can be determined. This method of measuring oxygen saturation has been shown to be quite accurate.[28–30] Ideally, pulse oximetry allows the gastrointestinal assistant and the endoscopist to detect hypoxemia before the patient experiences any adverse events. Pulse oximetry has several characteristics that make it ideal for monitoring patients during sedation and analgesia. It is simple to use, noninvasive, and portable; additionally, it does not interfere with the procedure, provides continuous monitoring, and has built-in alarms to alert the gastrointestinal assistant and endoscopist to abnormal measurements. Pulse oximetry has some limitations. Only 2 forms of hemoglobin may be identified (oxyhemoglobin and deoxyhemoglobin); in patients with dyshemoglobinemia (ie, methemoglobinemia), errors in oxygen saturation measurement may occur.[31–33] Additionally, the probe is easily dislodged, and a good pulse waveform is necessary to differentiate oxygen desaturation from artifact accurately. Pulse oximetry measurements are affected by decreased perfusion pressure (shock or vasoconstriction) and nail polish.

Measurement of heart rate, blood pressure, and electrocardiographic monitoring can be performed easily with available electronic monitor devices available today. These measurements are the standard of care in the United States. These variables should be measured before, during, and after endoscopy. Although physiologic changes in blood pressure, pulse, and cardiac rhythm occur during sedation and analgesia for endoscopic procedures, most of these physiologic changes do not result in clinically relevant adverse events.[34] Patients with significant cardiac disease are more likely to experience adverse events.[35] During and after sedation and analgesia, the patient's heart rate and cardiac rhythm should be monitored continuously. During routine endoscopic procedures, the blood pressure should be measured every 5 to 10 minutes. In more difficult endoscopic procedures and in patients with more severe comorbid disease, blood pressure should be monitored every 3 to 5 minutes. Clinical monitoring of the patient (oxygen saturation, blood pressure, heart rate, and electrocardiographic monitoring) must be continued throughout the recovery period (**Box 1**).

Significant carbon dioxide retention is a potential adverse event associated with sedation and analgesia. To date there are insufficient data to demonstrate improved clinical outcomes from the use of capnography in adults undergoing moderate sedation for gastrointestinal endoscopic procedures.[36] Therefore, routine use of capnography is not required during moderate sedation for gastrointestinal endoscopic procedures.[25]

Patients undergoing endoscopic procedures in an ambulatory endoscopy center can be discharged after an appropriate recovery period. A quantifiable set of discharge criteria must be met before discharging the patient. These criteria should include assessment of response to verbal stimuli, measurement of blood pressure and pulse, response to pain stimuli, presence of nausea or vomiting, and assessment of skin color. A modified Aldrete scoring system is used in the author's facility in Rockford, Ilinois, and is presented in **Table 5**. A score is calculated, and a required threshold score must be met before discharge. Verbal and written instructions should be provided to the patient, preferably in the presence of the responsible person escorting the patient. Although the immediate recovery from sedation and analgesia has been completed by the time of discharge, drugs may have lingering effects. Patients recovering from sedation and analgesia should not drive a car, operate machinery, or use alcohol for 24 hours. These restrictions still apply if flumazenil or naloxone has been administered.

Operations Management

Operations management provides the foundation for understanding how to operate and manage an efficient AEC.

Operations management deals with processes, those fundamental activities that organizations use to do work and achieve their goals.[37] A process is an event or activity that incorporates 1 or more events or activities and ultimately transforms them into an output for its customers. Successful operations management leads to efficiency. The term operations management refers to the systematic design, direction, and control of processes that transform inputs into services for internal as well as external customers.[37]

For an organization to operate efficiently, all employees must work together to complete the delivery of the service offered. Processes provide outputs, often services, to customers.[37] Customers include internal customers, internal suppliers, external customers, and external suppliers. Internal customers are employees who rely on inputs from other employees to perform their work (eg, schedulers, nurses, billing staff).[37] Internal suppliers are employees who supply important information or materials to a firm's processes (eg, accounting, information technology).[37] External customers are

---

Box 1
Guide for appropriate equipment in an ambulatory surgery center

- Uninterruptible power source
- Backup generator

Intravenous equipment

- Gloves
- Tourniquets
- Alcohol wipes
- Sterile gauze pads
- Intravenous catheters (needleless intravenous system preferred)
- Intravenous tubing
- Intravenous fluid
- Needles
- Various size syringes

Basic air management equipment

- Oxygen (tank with regulator)
- Suction
- Suction catheters
- Face masks
- Oral and nasal airways
- Self-inflating breathing bag (valve set)
- Lubricant

Advanced airway management equipment

- Laryngoscope handles (handles and blades)
- Endotracheal tubes
- Stylet

Emergency medications

- Atropine
- Glucose
- Epinephrine
- Lidocaine
- Diphenhydramine
- Hydrocortisone or methylprednisolone
- Diazepam or midazolam

Emergency cardiac cart (crash cart) for appropriately trained personnel

- Appropriately stocked
- Appropriately maintained

Table 5 Discharge criteria	
Assessment	**Score**
Patient is fully awake	2
Patient is arousable on calling	1
Patient is not responding	0
Blood Pressure 30 mm of baseline level	2
Blood Pressure 30–40 mm of baseline level	1
Blood Pressure >40 mm of baseline level	0
Able to deep breathe freely	2
Dyspneic or limited breathing	1
Apneic	0
Minimal to no pain or nausea	2
Moderate pain or vomiting	1
Severe pain or vomiting	0
Pink	2
Pale, dusky, blotchy, or other	1
Cyanotic	0
Total score for assessment (total needs to be 9 or 10)	

either intermediaries or end-users buying or using the final service offered by an organization (eg, referring physicians, patients).[37] Finally, external suppliers are businesses or individuals who provide resources, services, products, and materials for the organization's short-term and long-term needs (eg, pharmaceutical and endoscopy companies).[37] Organizational efficiency is directly related to the successful implementation of its processes. When processes are effective, organizational efficiency follows. Organizational efficiency leads to the delivery of services that are valued by customers. In the current health care environment, value as perceived by patients is best defined by the delivery of efficient and high-quality health care. In the near future, payers will also expect the delivery of efficient, high-quality health care services.

Efficiency in Endoscopy

Efficiency can be planned and assessed on multiple levels and in the context of many variables when delivering endoscopic services.[38] The physical environment of an endoscopy laboratory should be designed to allow for the efficient and safe movement of staff, patients, and family throughout the facility. Architects use flow diagrams to plan movement and flow throughout the facility (**Fig. 1**). Designers of the physical

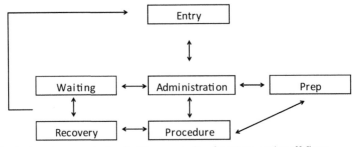

Fig. 1. Physical environment of a facility: example of patient and staff flow.

environment should obtain input from a team of administrators, physicians, and staff who best understand flow patterns through a facility. Their input is extremely important in arranging the flow relationships within an endoscopic facility and to maximize efficiency, minimize travel distance, and achieve economy of movement.[39] It is also important to consider space efficiency. Preparation, recovery, and endoscopic reprocessing rooms must be strategically located to allow for effective and efficient movement of patients, staff, and equipment to and from the endoscopy rooms. In successful endoscopy units, preparation, recovery, endoscopic reprocessing, and patient flow all occur efficiently and safely.

Throughput is defined as the movement of patients through a facility. Throughput maximizes use of space. Three factors greatly influence throughput: number of procedure rooms, number of preparation/recovery beds, and number of staff. There are no evidence-based data identifying the ideal number of endoscopy rooms. However, most experts agree that most efficient units use 3 to 4 endoscopy rooms. For every active endoscopy room, there should be a minimum of 3, and ideally 4, preparation/recovery beds.[40,41] This number of preparation/recovery beds avoids delay in performing endoscopy on the next patient.

The most important factor affecting throughput is staff number. There should be at least 1 staff member, typically a registered nurse, in each endoscopy room. Additionally, there should be a minimum of 2.5 full-time equivalents (FTEs) for preparation and recovery for each active endoscopy room. At Rockford Gastroenterology Associates (RGA), it has been found that a dedicated endoscope technician leads to more efficient room turnover. These technicians also assist with simple tasks during endoscopic procedures. When using dedicated endoscope technicians, one should plan on 0.5 to 0.75 FTEs per active endoscopy room. These recommendations represent minimum staffing levels. Each laboratory should identify and develop staffing ratios that best meet its needs.

Block scheduling is the most efficient way to schedule endoscopic procedures; it maximizes convenience for physicians and patients. Using standard time slots (30 minutes) for endoscopic procedures allows schedulers to offer patients more options when scheduling procedures. Block scheduling also offers flexibility regarding individual physician needs during endoscopy. For example, some physicians require more than the time allotted in standard slots. To accommodate such physicians, scheduling can arrange a more favorable ratio of esophagogastroduodenoscopy (EGDs) to colonoscopies or schedule 1 less procedure per block. This flexibility will help prevent delays in starting the procedure in the following block and allow for timely discharge of patients at the end of the day.

At RGA, 2 changes have recently been implemented in the scheduling process that have benefitted patients. RGA uses an alpha split (alphabetical scheduling by name) method to schedule patients. Each scheduler is responsible for a segment of the alphabet. Alpha split scheduling has led to more equal distribution of work among schedulers, consistency, accountability, and increased patient satisfaction through improved patient relationships. RGA also implemented a dedicated screening colonoscopy scheduler. This allows for better patient tracking, leading to more effective counseling for patients. Importantly, the conversion rate, defined as converting the initial request for colonoscopy into the patient completing the colonoscopic examination, to improve. Prior to implementation of a dedicated screening scheduler, the conversion rate was 55%. After implementation of this scheduler, the rate increased to 85%.

Open-access endoscopy has become common in the United States, primarily to accommodate the volume of screening procedures required by the healthy population.[38] Consultative care is not always necessary prior to performing endoscopic procedures. Open-access endoscopy should have strict criteria defining patient eligibility (for open-access procedures). Once criteria have been developed and implemented, it is important to share the guidelines with referring physicians so they better understand which patients are eligible for open-access endoscopy. Also, the criteria are used by nursing staff to help screen appropriate patients for open-access endoscopy and avoid inappropriate patient scheduling. The goal of open-access endoscopy is to increase patient convenience while maintaining quality care.

Open-access endoscopy has benefits for the cognitive aspect of a practice. By offering open-access endoscopy to healthy patients, thereby avoiding unnecessary clinic visits, more slots for consultative services will be available to patients with active gastrointestinal problems. Patients who participate in open-access endoscopy rarely require subsequent consultative services and typically are compliant with the endoscopist's recommendations regarding follow-up care.

SUMMARY

The most successful AECs will navigate the dynamic changes in the health care system by defining safe and efficient care. Physician and administrative leadership will need to understand and implement the topics discussed in the article to optimize safety, meet patient expectations, and manage an efficient AEC.

REFERENCES

1. Daneshmend TK, Bell GD, Logan RF. Sedation for upper gastrointestinal endoscopy: results of a nationwide survey. Gut 1991;32:12–5.
2. Keeffe EB, O'Connor KW. 1989 ASGE Survey of endoscopic sedation in monitoring practices. Gastrointest Endosc 1990;36:S13–8.
3. Standards of Practice Committee of the American Society for Gastrointestinal Endoscopy, Lichtenstein DR, Jagannath S, Baron TH, et al. Sedation and anesthesia in GI endoscopy. Gastrointest Endosc 2008;68(5):815–26.
4. American Society of Anesthesiologists Task Force on Sedation and Analgesia by Non-Anesthesiologists. Practice guidelines for sedation and analgesia by non-anesthesiologists. Anesthesiology 2002;96(4):1004–17.
5. Liu H, Waxman DA, Main R, et al. Utilization of anesthesia services during outpatient endoscopies and colonoscopies and associated spending in 2003-2009. JAMA 2012;307(11):1178–84.
6. Diab FH, King PD, Barthel JS, et al. Efficacy and safety of combined meperidine and midazolam for EGD sedation compared with midazolam alone. Am J Gastroenterol 1996;91(6):1120–5.
7. Froehlich F, Thorens J, Schwizer W, et al. Sedation and analgesia for colonoscopy: patient tolerance, pain, and cardiorespiratory parameters. Gastrointest Endosc 1997;45(1):1–9.
8. Ginsberg GG, Lewis JH, Gallagher JE, et al. Diazepam versus midazolam for colonoscopy: a prospective evaluation of predicted versus actual dosing requirements. Gastrointest Endosc 1992;38(6):651–6.
9. Martin JP, Arlett PA, Holdstock G. Development of a sedation policy for upper GI endoscopy based on an audit of patients' perception of the procedure. Eur J Gastroenterol Hepatol 1996;8(4):355–7.
10. Bell GD. Review article: premedication and intravenous sedation for upper gastrointestinal endoscopy. Aliment Pharmacol Ther 1990;4(2):103–22.

11. Freeman ML. Sedation and monitoring for gastrointestinal endoscopy. In: Yamada T, editor. Textbook of gastroenterology, vol. 2, 3rd edition. Philadelphia: Lippincott Williams & Wilkins; 1999. p. 26–64.

12. Arrowsmith JB, Gerstman BB, Fleischer DE, et al. Results from the American Society for Gastrointestinal Endoscopy/U.S. Food and Drug Administration collaborative study on complication rates and drug use during gastrointestinal endoscopy. Gastrointest Endosc 1991;37(4):421–7.

13. Ben- Shlomo I, abd-el-Khalim H, Ezry J, et al. Midazolam acts synergistically with fentanyl for induction of anaesthesia. Br J Anaesth 1990;64(1):45–7.

14. Halliday NJ, Dundee JW, Harper KW. Influence of fentanyl and alfentanil pretreatment of the action of midazolam. Br J Anaesth 1985;54:935–9.

15. Froehlich F, Schwizer W, Thorens J, et al. Conscious sedation for gastroscopy: patient tolerance and cardiorespiratory parameters. Gastroenterology 1995; 108:697–704.

16. Nagengast RM. Sedation and monitoring in gastrointestinal endoscopy. Scand J Gastroenterol 1993;28:28–32.

17. Marinella JA. Propofol for sedation in the intensive care unit: essentials for the clinician. Respir Med 1997;91:505–10.

18. Thompson AM, Park KGM, Kerr F, et al. Safety of fiberoptic endoscopy: analysis of cardio-respiratory events. Br J Surg 1992;79:1046–9.

19. Carlsson U, Grattidge P. Sedation for upper gastrointestinal endoscopy: a comparative study of propofol and midazolam. Endoscopy 1995;27:240–3.

20. Patterson KW, Casey PB, Murray JP, et al. Propofol sedation for outpatient upper gastrointestinal endoscopy: comparison with midazolam. Br J Anaesth 1991;67: 108–11.

21. Vargo JJ, Zuccaro G, Dumot JA, et al. Gastroenterologist-administered propofol for therapeutic upper endoscopy with graphic assessment of respiratory activity: a case series. Gastrointest Endosc 2000;52:250–5.

22. Roseveare C, Seavell C, Patel P, et al. Patient-controlled sedation and analgesia, using propofol and alfentanil during colonoscopy: a perspective randomized trial. Endoscopy 1998;30:768–73.

23. Rosario MT, Costa NF. Combination of midazolam and flumazenil in upper gastrointestinal endoscopy, a double-blind randomized study. Gastrointest Endosc 1990;36:30–3.

24. Saletin M, Malchow H, Muhlhofer H, et al. A randomized controlled trial to evaluate the effects of flumazenil after midazolam premedication in outpatients undergoing colonoscopy. Endoscopy 1991;23:31–3.

25. ASGE Ensuring Safety in the Gastrointestinal Endoscopy Unit Task Force, Calderwood AH, Chapman FJ, et al. Guidelines for safety in the gastrointestinal endoscopy unit. Gastrointest Endosc 2014;79(3):363–72.

26. Cooper GS, Blades EW. Indications, contraindications, and complications of upper gastrointestinal endoscopy. In: Sivak MV Jr, editor. Gastroenterologic endoscopy. 2nd edition. Philadelphia: WB Saunders; 1999. p. 438–54.

27. Gander JS. Guideline for isolation precautions in hospitals. Hospital Infection Control Practices Advisory Committee. Infect Control Hosp Epidemiol 1996;17: 53–80.

28. Alexander CM, Tella LE, Gross JB. Principles of pulse oximetry: theoretical and practical considerations. Anesth Analg 1989;68:368–76.

29. The use of pulse oximetry during conscious sedation. Council on ScientificAffairs, American Medical Association. JAMA 1993;270:1463–8.

30. Rempter KK, Barker SJ. Pulse oximetry. Anesthesiology 1989;70:98–108.

31. Eisenkraft JB. Carboxy hemoglobin and pulse oximetry. Anesthesiology 1988;68: 300–1.
32. Taylor MB, Whitman JG. The current status of pulse oximetry. Anesthesiology 1986;41:943–9.
33. Visco DM, Tolpin E, Straughn JC, et al. Arterial oxygen saturation in sedated patients undergoing gastrointestinal endoscopy and a review of pulse oximetry. Del Med J 1989;61:533–42.
34. Fennerty MB, Earnest DL, Hudson PB, et al. Physiologic changes during colonoscopy. Gastrointest Endosc 1990;36:22–5.
35. Leiberman DA, Wuerker CK, Caton RM. Cardiopulmonary risk of EGD: role of endoscope diameter and systemic sedation. Gastroenterology 1985;88:468–72.
36. Multi-Society Statement: universal adoption of capnography for moderate sedation in adults undergoing upper endoscopy and colonoscopy has not been shown to improve patient safety or clinical outcomes and significantly increases costs for moderate sedation. 2012. Available at: http://www.asge.org/uploadedFiles/Publications_(public)/Practice_guidelines/Endoscopy_premalignant_malignant_conditions.pdf. Accessed December 8, 2015.
37. Krajewski LJ. Operations management: processes and value chains. Upper Saddle River (NJ): Pearson Prentice Hall; 2007.
38. Petersen BT. Promoting efficiency in gastrointestinal endoscopy. Gastrointest Endosc Clin N Am 2006;16:671–85.
39. Frakes JT. Setting up an endoscopic facility. In: Ginsberg GG, Kochman ML, Norton ID, et al, editors. Clinical gastrointestinal endoscopy. London: Elsevier Science; 2005. p. 13–27.
40. Yong E, Zenkova O, Saibil F, et al. Efficiency of an endoscopy suite in a teaching hospital: delays, prolonged procedures, and hospital waiting times. Gastrointest Endosc 2006;64:760–4.
41. Marus SN. Efficiency in endoscopy centers. Gastrointest Endosc 2006;64:765–7.

Quality Assurance in the Endoscopy Suite
Sedation and Monitoring

Zachary P. Harris, MD[a], Julia Liu, MD, MSc, FACG, FACP, FASGE[a],
John R. Saltzman, MD[b],*

KEYWORDS

- Moderate sedation • Propofol • Colonoscopy • Quality • Endoscopy safety
- Procedural sedation

KEY POINTS

- Preprocedure assessment includes proper informed consent, a history and physical examination, risk assessment, a sedation plan, and a team pause or time-out.
- Intraprocedure time begins with sedation and ends with removal of the endoscope and includes guideline-based patient monitoring and complication management.
- The postprocedure assessment includes established discharge criteria, proper patient instructions, tracking of adverse events, and collection of patient satisfaction scores.
- Competency in procedural sedation includes formal training and education in sedation, an understanding of the pharmacokinetics and pharmacodynamics of sedation agents, and proper endoscopic personnel.

INTRODUCTION

With the rapid growth of endoscopic procedures, particularly in screening of colon cancer, the importance of patient tolerance and safety while conducting these procedures has also increased. Important for optimal performance and quality outcomes are a variety of medications for sedation and analgesia. Endoscopic sedation has traditionally included a benzodiazepine, most commonly midazolam, and an opioid analgesic, usually fentanyl. Propofol is an increasingly used sedative option through a variety of administration modalities and personnel. While the utility of the different sedation options and newer sedation modalities are explored, it is imperative that good quality-assurance measures be followed and competency maintained.

Disclosure: The authors have nothing to disclose.
[a] Department of Medicine, University of Arkansas for Medical Sciences, 4301 West Markham Street, Little Rock, AR 72205, USA; [b] Brigham and Women's Hospital, Harvard Medical School, 75 Francis Street, Boston, MA 02115, USA
* Corresponding author.
E-mail address: jsaltzman@bwh.harvard.edu

Gastrointest Endoscopy Clin N Am 26 (2016) 553–562
http://dx.doi.org/10.1016/j.giec.2016.02.008
1052-5157/16/$ – see front matter © 2016 Elsevier Inc. All rights reserved.

This article reviews the endoscopic sedation and monitoring quality initiatives and guidelines in the current literature.

QUALITY-ASSURANCE COMPETENCIES
Preprocedure Assessment

Before the endoscopic procedure, it is imperative that the safety of the patient be considered. Safety in endoscopic sedation can be categorized into several components, including but not limited to patient risk assessment, informed consent, monitoring compliance, training/education, and adverse event tracking.[1,2] In addition, the American Society for Gastrointestinal Endoscopy (ASGE) recommends measuring preprocedure safety by how frequently certain issues are addressed, including informed consent, completion and documentation of a history and physical examination, risk assessment, development of a sedation plan, and performance of team pause or time-out.[3] The essential steps for preprocedure assessment are discussed here.

Informed consent

Informed consent is a crucial component of all endoscopic procedures and adheres to the medical ethical principle of patient autonomy. It allows patients to be involved in their own care and creates the opportunity for each patient to ask questions and assist in decision making. With the exception of some emergent procedures, every attempt should be made to obtain and document proper informed consent before diagnostic and therapeutic endoscopic interventions. The discussion should include the sedation plan as well as the benefits and risks of sedation. Benefits include patient comfort and improvement of diagnostic procedure performance and therapeutic yield. Important risks include unintended deeper levels of sedation, suppression of respiration, postoperative somnolence, aspiration, and adverse reactions to sedation medications. Furthermore, the clinician who administers the sedation should personally obtain consent for sedation, and this should be done separately if the endoscopist will not be the sedation provider.

There does not seem to be any consensus on the exact timing and location for obtaining informed consent. However, the consent should ideally be obtained when there is sufficient time to explain and answer all questions in an environment that is comfortable for the patient.

History and physical examination

Each patient should undergo an assessment of medications, medical problems, and allergies, and a focused physical examination before sedation and endoscopy. This process should be done before the endoscopic procedure and thus should be separate from the endoscopy report. There should be a focus on identifying the potential complications from sedation and endoscopy, as well as the indications for the selected sedation. Specific history points that should be emphasized include previous sedation reactions (including both personal and family history of reactions to anesthesia), medication allergies, and potential medication interactions. Social history should incorporate any history of tobacco, alcohol, or substance use or abuse.

Risk assessment

Before sedation and endoscopy begins, each patient should be risk stratified to identify potential complications and adverse events. Objective methods such as the American Society of Anesthesiologists (ASA) score should be used to guide the sedation plan; this includes whether it is safe to proceed with the current plan with or without modifications and can be used as a screening tool for sedation.

The ASA score is a subjective assessment of a patient's overall health and is based on 6 classes (I to VI):

I. A normal healthy patient
II. A patient with mild systemic disease
III. A patient with severe systemic disease
IV. A patient with severe systemic disease that is a constant threat to life
V. A moribund patient who is not expected to survive without the operation
VI. A declared brain-dead patient whose organs are being removed for donor purposes[4,5]

Sedation plan

Development and documentation of a sedation plan is required before beginning endoscopic procedures. Intended levels of sedation are categorized as no sedation, minimal sedation, moderate sedation, deep sedation, and general anesthesia.

- Minimal sedation that provides anxiolysis refers to a drug-induced state during which patients respond normally to verbal commands. Cognitive function and coordination may be impaired, but ventilatory and cardiovascular functions are unaffected.
- Moderate sedation (also commonly called intravenous conscious sedation) refers to a drug-induced depression of consciousness during which patients respond purposefully to verbal commands, either alone or accompanied by light tactile stimulation. No interventions are required to maintain a patent airway, and ventilation is spontaneous and adequate. Cardiovascular function is maintained. Moderate sedation is often used to perform endoscopic procedures.
- Deep sedation refers to drug-induced depression of consciousness during which patients cannot easily be aroused, but respond purposefully following repeated or painful stimulation. The ability to independently maintain ventilatory function may be impaired. Patients may require assistance in maintaining a patent airway, and spontaneous ventilation may be inadequate. Cardiovascular function is usually maintained. Deep sedation is also commonly used during endoscopic procedures, especially when propofol is used.
- General anesthesia refers to a drug-induced loss of consciousness during which patients are not arousable, even by painful stimulation. The ability to independently maintain ventilatory function is impaired. Such patients often require assistance in maintaining a patent airway, and positive pressure ventilation may be required because of depressed spontaneous ventilation or drug-induced depression of neuromuscular function. Cardiovascular function may be impaired.[6] General anesthesia is less frequently used in general endoscopy, although it is often used in complex endoscopic procedures such as endoscopic retrograde cholangiopancreatography.

Physicians should be familiar with each level of sedation but should also be aware that these are levels of sedation within a spectrum. Physicians administering sedation to an intended level should also be trained for and comfortable with rescue methods, in the event that the patient enters a deeper than intended state of sedation.

Team pause

Also known as a time-out, the team pause is part of good patient care and is mandated by most national accrediting bodies, including the Joint Commission as well as the Centers for Medicare and Medicaid Services. The team pause should always be performed before initiation of sedation or insertion of the endoscope. During the team pause, patients should be asked to state their name and date of birth. The answer should be compared with the patient's name band and verified with any documentation in the room, including the consent form, electronic medical health record, and the endoscopy reporting system.[7] The procedure being performed should be noted and any specific equipment or concerns discussed. Any patient allergies should also be mentioned. The need for antibiotics or anticipated blood loss should also be noted when applicable. The team pause should be documented in the medical record. The team pause should be repeated if a new team member enters the procedure room after the initial team pause is complete.

Intraprocedure Assessment

Intraprocedure time begins with either sedation or insertion of the endoscope and lasts until the sedation is complete and the endoscope is removed. The administration and documentation of medications, frequency of reversal agent use, and rate of early termination because of adverse sedation issues are all integral quality indicators.[3]

Monitoring

For the duration of the procedure, cardiopulmonary monitoring should be used to minimize adverse events. ASGE and ASA guidelines include use of pulse rate, blood pressure, and oximetry. The ASA also recommends continuous electrocardiography for patients with significant cardiovascular disease or dysrhythmias.[5] Both ASGE and ASA guidelines recommend that capnography be considered for patients receiving deep sedation; however, only the ASA recommends using capnography for all patients undergoing moderate sedation. The ASGE states that there are insufficient data to mandate its use in all patients undergoing endoscopy with moderate sedation.[8–10] Nevertheless, after publication of the ASA guidelines many endoscopy suites routinely include capnography monitoring. Transcutaneous capnometry to measure carbon dioxide has also been shown to prevent severe carbon dioxide retention more effectively than intensive clinical monitoring and pulse oximetry alone.[11] Although not shown in controlled trials of endoscopy, it is generally thought that these monitoring modalities improve patient safety.

Complication management

Complications during endoscopy, although infrequent, are often related to the sedation rather than the endoscopic procedure. Complications from endoscopic sedation include phlebitis from intravenous benzodiazepine administration, hypoxemia, cardiac arrhythmias, and aspiration. The most common and serious complications are cardiopulmonary. Reversal agents are used to move patients to a lower level of sedation, typically when patients become oversedated and hypoxic. Naloxone is used to reverse the sedation and respiratory depression caused by opioids. Although flumazenil is used to reverse the sedation caused by benzodiazepines, it tends to have little effect on respiratory depression; because of this, naloxone should generally be given before flumazenil in the case of respiratory depression in a patient who has received both an opioid and a benzodiazepine for sedation. Caution should be used in patients who chronically take benzodiazepines, certain antidepressants, or antiepileptics because flumazenil administration can lower the seizure threshold. Of note, propofol has no currently available antagonist. It is important to recognize that the half-lives of the reversal agents are generally much shorter than the half-lives of the sedative agent being reversed. Thus patients need to be monitored after reversal until the effect of the sedative has worn off and for a minimum of 90 minutes.

At best there is negligible evidence in current literature to support the elective use of reversal agents to decrease recovery time and thus this elective use is not recommended.[12] It is unclear whether there are cost-savings that are not outweighed by the cost of the routine use of these agents. Further, the issue of shorter half-lives of the reversal agents than the sedative agents could lead to resedation and possible complications.

Hypoxemia is common during endoscopic sedation. Moreover, some studies have shown a degree of hypoxemia in patients undergoing endoscopic procedures, even in those who are not sedated.[13] Routine use of supplemental oxygen is recommended, especially in patients with risk factors for hypoxemia, which include above average endoscopic sedation dose administration, longer procedure times (eg, endoscopic ultrasonography), and patients with underlying cardiopulmonary disease. In addition, there may be a correlation with desaturation and arrhythmias, further supporting the benefits of routine supplemental oxygen use.[14]

Postprocedure Assessment

The postprocedure period is typically defined as the time span from when the endoscope is removed to the first follow-up. Established discharge criteria should be met before each patient is allowed to leave, discharge instructions should be provided, adverse events should be documented, and patient satisfaction should be evaluated.

Discharge criteria
Every endoscopy center should have a preset list of criteria that must be met before patient discharge after endoscopy. There are 2 established grading systems that assess readiness for phase II recovery and home, respectively, that have been determined to be as safe as clinical assessment and facilitate faster discharge times: the Aldrete Scoring System (**Table 1**) and the Postanesthetic Discharge Scoring System (**Table 2**).[15,16] If reversal agents were used, monitoring for at least 90 minutes after administration is recommended for signs of resedation. Although antagonist duration lasts approximately 1 hour, midazolam duration can last up to 80 minutes.

Patient instructions
Before discharge, patients should be provided with written discharge instructions that include diet and activity restrictions if applicable, any medication changes, explanation of biopsy results (or details of how biopsy notification will be communicated), contact information for questions and emergencies, and follow-up appointment information. Signs and symptoms of delayed adverse events should also be provided as well as instructions to call a physician in the event of an adverse event.

Adverse events
All endoscopy centers should have a tracking system in place to monitor and document any adverse event that occurred from the beginning of endoscopy to the end of the postprocedure period. Each event should be classified according to level of severity, timing, and the level of liability attributable to the sedation, endoscopic procedure, and the patient. Aborted procedures and administration of reversal agents do not need to be automatically classified as adverse events. This process should be done in a nonpunitive manner to encourage reporting of these events in the context of continuous quality improvement. Regular meetings of staff, including physicians and nurses, to review all adverse events are an important aspect of quality assurance.

Patient satisfaction
Patient satisfaction should be collected if feasible and recorded by using a standardized questionnaire. The ASGE recommends the use of the GHAA-9 (Group Health

Table 1 The Aldrete Scoring System	
Respiration	
Ability to cough and breathe deeply	2
Dyspneic or limited breathing	1
Apneic	0
Blood Pressure	
±20% of preanesthesia level	2
±20%–50% of preanesthesia level	1
± >50% preanesthesia level, or requiring pharmacologic intervention	0
Color (or Oxygen Saturation)	
Pink and normal (or oxygen saturation >92%)	2
Pale, dusky, blotched (or needs oxygen to maintain saturation >90%)	1
Cyanotic (or oxygen saturation <90% with oxygen)	0
Consciousness	
Awake and oriented × 3	2
Arousable to command	1
Not responding	0
Activity	
Ability to move all 4 extremities on command	2
Ability to move 2 extremities on command	1
Ability to move 0 extremities on command	0
Patients with score ≥8 for 2 consecutive measurements are considered fit for discharge home	Total score (0–10)

Association of America 9) patient satisfaction questionnaire modified for use after endoscopy (**Fig. 1**).[3,17]

COMPETENCY IN ENDOSCOPIC SEDATION
Training

Any physician who oversees the administration of sedation medications should undergo formal training and education in sedation. According to the Multisociety Sedation Curriculum for Gastrointestinal Endoscopy (MSCGE), training should focus on medical knowledge related to the available sedation agents, identifying indications and contraindications, principles of airway management, consent process, professionalism, and personal communication skills. These items should ideally be evaluated through a combination of direct observation of hands-on training and simulation labs (if available) during gastroenterology fellowship training, Web-based simulations, written examinations, patient satisfaction surveys, and chart audit/reviews. Furthermore, the MSCGE defines principles of training assessment as follows:

1. Assessment should be linked to learning goals and completion of learning modules.
2. Learning environment and evaluation should be of high quality.
3. Evaluation should be timely, reliable, transparent, engaging, and efficient.[16]

Pharmacology

Before endoscopy training, trainees should possess a full understanding of the pharmacokinetics and pharmacodynamics of sedation agents, including drug interactions and

Table 2
Modified Postanesthetic Discharge Scoring System

Vital Signs	
BP and HR ±20% of preendoscopy value	2
BP and HR ±20%–40% of preendoscopy value	1
BP and HR ±40% of preendoscopy value	0
Activity	
Steady gait, no dizziness, or meets preendoscopy level	2
Requires assistance	1
Unable to ambulate	0
Nausea and Vomiting	
No or minimal/treated with PO medication	2
Moderate/treated with parenteral medication	1
Severe/continues despite treatment	0
Pain	
Minimal or no pain (numerical analogue scale = 0–3)	2
Moderate (numerical analogue scale = 4–6)	1
Severe (numerical analogue scale = 7–10)	0
Surgical Bleeding	
None or minimal (not requiring intervention)	2
Moderate (1 episode of hematemesis or rectal bleeding)	1
Severe (≥2 episodes of hematemesis or rectal bleeding)	0
Patients with score ≥9 for 2 consecutive measurements are considered fit for discharge home	Total score (0–10)

Abbreviations: BP, blood pressure; HR, heart rate; PO, by mouth.

potential adverse effects. They should then acquire skill in administering each available medication through direct supervision. Simulation tests, if available, may be used before beginning training in the endoscopy suite. Physicians should be comfortable with the levels of sedation for which they aim and should also be proficient in rescue methods and reversal agents in the event that the patient reaches a deeper than intended level of sedation or, alternatively, another type of adverse reaction occurs.

In terms of your satisfaction, how would you rate each of the following:

1. How long you waited to get an appointment.

Excellent	Very good	Good	Fair	Poor

2. Length of time spent waiting for the procedure.

Excellent	Very good	Good	Fair	Poor

3. The personal manner (courtesy, respect, sensitivity, friendliness) of the physician who performed your procedure.

Excellent	Very good	Good	Fair	Poor

4. The technical skills (thoroughness, carefulness, competence) of the physician who performed your procedure.

Excellent	Very good	Good	Fair	Poor

5. The personal manner (courtesy, respect, sensitivity, friendliness) of the nurses and the other support staff.

Excellent	Very good	Good	Fair	Poor

6. Adequacy of explanation of what was done for you—all your questions answered.

Excellent	Very good	Good	Fair	Poor

7. Overall rating of the visit

Excellent	Very good	Good	Fair	Poor

Fig. 1. The modified GHAA-9 assessment of patient satisfaction.

Although there has been the widespread practice of endoscopy without sedation internationally, most guidelines recommend the use of sedation for patients undergoing gastrointestinal endoscopy.[18] Traditionally, benzodiazepines with opioids have been used. However, use of propofol for gastrointestinal endoscopy sedation may be both patient centered and economical for the endoscopy center, primarily through increased patient satisfaction and by facilitating quicker patient turnover. Overall cost benefits are not as clear and vary widely depending on the modality and personnel used to administer propofol.[19]

Personnel

Although propofol is widely used as a gastrointestinal endoscopy sedation agent, who and how it should be administered remain topics of debate. There are 2 major types of personnel settings: (1) a nurse trained in endoscopic sedation administering propofol under the direction of the endoscopist, which is termed endoscopist-directed sedation; (2) propofol directly administered and monitored by an anesthesia-trained physician or nurse anesthetist, known as monitored anesthesia care (MAC). The product label for propofol seems to reserve its use in general anesthesia or monitored sedation by persons trained in the administration of general anesthesia; however, there are a large number of studies that support the safety and efficacy of endoscopist-directed sedation. Many gastroenterologists think that the label should be changed to allow for nonanesthesiologist propofol sedation administration.[19–22] Cohen and colleagues[6] surmised that further outcome studies comparing MAC with endoscopist-directed sedation need to be performed. Rex and colleagues[23] further speculated that, because of the large financial incentives from special interest groups, MAC will continue to be the major personnel modality for propofol administration for gastrointestinal endoscopy sedation.

Other propofol delivery systems are currently under investigation, most notably computer assisted delivery. The SEDAYSYS (Ethicon Endo-Surgery) system has US Food and Drug Administration approval, although it may be still considered experimental, and was just voluntarily withdrawn by the company and thus is not currently available. It consists of 2 major components: a drug delivery system and a patient monitoring system. The self-contained system uses a patient earpiece and handheld device as well as cardiopulmonary monitoring as real-time feedback to adjust drug delivery.[24]

SUMMARY

Quality measures and competency training are essential to ensure the safety of sedation in endoscopy. Comprehensive and safe endoscopic sedation is key to the success of gastrointestinal endoscopy. As progress continues in gastrointestinal endoscopy, systematic review, assessment, and directed updates of sedation quality measures will continue to be paramount. Further frameworks need to be provided and updated as outcome studies are published, particularly for propofol administration, and should be based on a multisociety consensus that is congruent with current legal precedent and good clinical practice.

REFERENCES

1. Armstrong D, Barkun A, Bridges R, et al. Canadian Association of Gastroenterology consensus guidelines on safety and quality indicators in endoscopy. Can J Gastroenterol 2012;26(1):17–31.
2. Allen JI. Quality assurance for gastrointestinal endoscopy. Curr Opin Gastroenterol 2012;28(5):442–50.

3. Rizk MK, Sawhney MS, Cohen J, et al. Quality indicators common to all GI endoscopic procedures. Gastrointest Endosc 2015;81(1):3–16.

4. Committee on Standards and Practice Parameters, Apfelbaum JL, Connis RT, Nickinovich DG, et al. Practice advisory for preanesthesia evaluation: an updated report by the American Society of Anesthesiologists Task Force on Preanesthesia Evaluation. Anesthesiology 2012;116:522.

5. American Society of Anesthesiologists Task Force on Sedation and Analgesia by Non-Anesthesiologists. Practice guidelines for sedation and analgesia by non-anesthesiologists. Anesthesiology 2002;96:1004–17.

6. Cohen LB, Delegge MH, Aisenberg J, et al. AGA Institute review of endoscopic sedation. Gastroenterology 2007;133:675–701.

7. Matharoo M, Thomas-Gibson S, Haycock A, et al. Implementation of an endoscopy safety checklist. Frontline Gastroenterol 2014;5:260–5.

8. ASGE Ensuring Safety in the Gastrointestinal Endoscopy Unit Task Force, Calderwood AH, Chapman FJ, et al. Guidelines for safety in the gastrointestinal endoscopy unit. Gastrointest Endosc 2014;79:363.

9. Beitz A, Riphaus A, Meining A, et al. Capnographic monitoring reduces the incidence of arterial oxygen desaturation and hypoxemia during propofol sedation for colonoscopy: a randomized, controlled study (ColoCap Study). Am J Gastroenterol 2012;107:1205.

10. Qadeer MA, Vargo JJ, Dumot JA, et al. Capnographic monitoring of respiratory activity improves safety of sedation for endoscopic cholangiopancreatography and ultrasonography. Gastroenterology 2009;136:1568.

11. Nelson DB, Freeman ML, Silvis SE, et al. A randomized, controlled trial of transcutaneous carbon dioxide monitoring during ERCP. Gastrointest Endosc 2000;51:288.

12. Chang AC, Solinger MA, Yang DT, et al. Impact of flumazenil on recovery after outpatient endoscopy: a placebo-controlled trial. Gastrointest Endosc 1999;49:573.

13. Yen D, Hu SC, Chen LS, et al. Arterial oxygen desaturation during emergent nonsedated upper gastrointestinal endoscopy in the emergency department. Am J Emerg Med 1997;15:644.

14. Lieberman DA, Wuerker CK, Katon RM. Cardiopulmonary risk of esophagogastroduodenoscopy. Role of endoscope diameter and systemic sedation. Gastroenterology 1985;88:468.

15. Trevisani L, Cifalà V, Gilli G, et al. Post-anaesthetic discharge scoring system to assess patient recovery and discharge after colonoscopy. World J Gastrointest Endosc 2013;5(10):502–7.

16. Vargo JJ, Delegge MH, Feld AD, et al. Multisociety sedation curriculum for gastrointestinal endoscopy. Gastrointest Endosc 2012;76:e1–25.

17. Johanson JF, Schmitt CM, Deas TM Jr, et al. Quality and outcomes assessment in gastrointestinal endoscopy. Gastrointest Endosc 2000;52:827–30.

18. Fanti L, Pier AT. Sedation and analgesia in gastrointestinal endoscopy: what's new? World J Gastroenterol 2010;16(20):2451–7.

19. Cohen LB, Benson AA. Issues in endoscopic sedation. Gastroenterol Hepatol 2009;5(8):565–70.

20. Vargo JJ, Bramley TJ, Meyer K, et al. Practice efficiency and economics. The case for rapid recovery sedation agents for colonoscopy in a screening population. J Clin Gastroenterol 2007;41:591–8.

21. Diprivan injectable emulsion [package insert]. AstraZeneca; 2005.

22. Rex DK, Heuss LT, Walker JA, et al. Trained registered nurses/endoscopy teams can administer propofol safely for endoscopy. Gastroenterology 2005;129:1384–91.

23. Rex DK, Deenadayalu V, Eid E. Gastroenterologist-directed propofol: an update. Gastrointest Endosc Clin North Am 2008;18:717–25, ix.
24. Pambianco DJ, Pruitt RE, Hardi R, et al. Computer-assisted personalized sedation system to administer propofol versus standard of care sedation for colonoscopy and EGD: a 1000 subject randomized, controlled, multi-center, pivotal trial. Gastroenterology 2008;135:294.

Computer-Assisted and Patient-Controlled Sedation Platforms

Daniel Pambianco, MD[a],*, Paul Niklewski, PhD[b,c,d]

KEYWORDS

- Sedation platforms • Computer-assisted sedation • Patient-controlled sedation
- Endoscopic sedation

KEY POINTS

- Ideal sedation requirements for endoscopy need to be matched to patient comfort, co-morbidity risks, procedural discomfort, and the length of the procedure in order to minimize the unnecessary risk of deeper sedation or general anesthesia.
- Most patients require moderate sedation for relatively short procedures for which the ideal agent or administration model is still being sought.
- Patient- and computer-controlled sedation have the ability to impact the quality and safety of sedation for endoscopic procedures.

INTRODUCTION

Endoscopic procedures are vitally important in maintaining the health of a patient population; however, these procedures are invasive and cause patient discomfort and anxiety. Sedation has become a necessary part of the endoscopic procedure to ensure patient compliance through patient comfort. Optimally, sedation requirements for endoscopy need to be matched to patient comfort, comorbidity risks, the anticipated procedural discomfort, and the length of the procedure in order to minimize the unnecessary risk of deeper sedation or general anesthesia.[1] Most patients require moderate sedation for relatively short procedures for which the ideal agent or administration model is still being sought.

Patient- and computer-controlled sedation have been long studied, more than 50 years; but these platforms are not yet accepted broadly as a means of sedation

[a] Charlottesville Medical Research, 325 Winding River Lane, Suite 102, Charlottesville, VA 22911, USA; [b] Department of Pharmacology and Cell Biophysics, University of Cincinnati College of Medicine, 231 Albert Sabin Way, University of Cincinnati, Cincinnati, OH 45267-0575, USA; [c] Xavier University, 3800 Victory Pkwy, Cincinnati, OH 45207, USA; [d] Sedasys, a Division of Ethicon Endo-Surgery, Inc, Ethicon Endo-Surgery Inc, 4545 Creek Road, Cincinnati, OH 45242, USA
* Corresponding author.
E-mail address: dpambianco@aol.com

Gastrointest Endoscopy Clin N Am 26 (2016) 563–576
http://dx.doi.org/10.1016/j.giec.2016.02.003
1052-5157/16/$ – see front matter © 2016 Elsevier Inc. All rights reserved.

giendo.theclinics.com

in the United States.[2,3] As these technologies have advanced, so has the ability to impact the quality and safety of sedation for endoscopic procedures. A review of the current state of these technologic advances is discussed.

SEDATION MEDICATIONS APPROPRIATE FOR COMPUTER AND PATIENT CONTROL

When selecting sedation agents for computer or patient control, the pharmacokinetic/pharmacodynamic (PK/PD) properties of the agent are paramount. Agents, such as midazolam, are less than ideal for infusions and computer or patient control, primarily because of their long onset and offset time. **Fig. 1** shows theoretic plasma and effect site concentrations for a single bolus dose of midazolam. As can be seen, the effect site concentration is not at steady state until almost 10 minutes. This time frame prohibits the ability to titrate for endoscopy procedures, especially those that last less than 10 minutes, such as esophagogastroduodenoscopy (EGD).

In recent years propofol has become the preferred sedative because of its PK/PD properties, allowing for rapid onset/offset and rapid clear-headed recovery. Propofol, when titrated, allows for a rapid and steady state titration. Propofol has historically been considered a general anesthetic, as it has been used to induce a state of general anesthesia. However, when titrated, it can be used for sedation. **Fig. 2** shows 3 plots of propofol infusion, all having a total of 187.5 mg delivered after 20 minutes. The top subplot shows a single bolus of propofol, with a maximum effect site concentration of approximately 6 µg/mL, a general anesthetic concentration. When that same amount of propofol is delivered in 4 boluses, the effect site concentration is significantly reduced to just more than 2 µg/mL, as shown in the middle subplot. The bottom subplot shows a steady state infusion, a preferred delivery method for sedation. In this case, a loading dose is delivered followed by a steady state delivery. Therefore, the peaks and valleys are managed, and the effect site concentration does not exceed approximately 1.5 µg/mL. The dose, and the method of delivery, defines the effect site concentration. Computer-controlled sedation allows for an increased degree of control of drug optimization, providing a potentially more stable sedation experience compared with traditional bolus dosing.

Using a drug such as propofol allows for procedural titration not possible with a drug such as midazolam, with a more significant onset/offset time. **Fig. 3** (scale

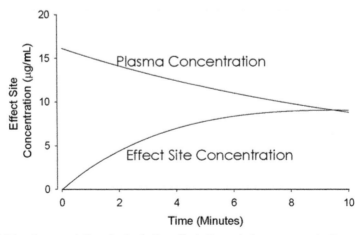

Fig. 1. Midazolam onset time for both the effect site and plasma concentration.

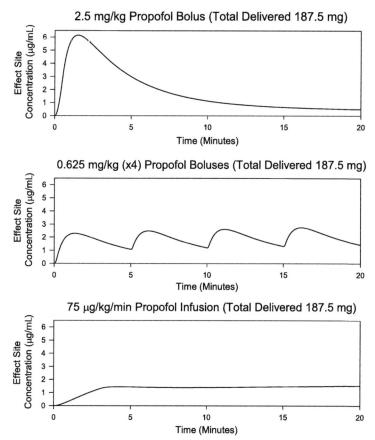

Fig. 2. Example of bolus dosing compared with infusion with a loading dose. Top subplot is a single bolus of propofol. The middle subplot shows 4 boluses distributed over the same time, with the same total propofol delivered. The bottom subplot shows a loading dose associated with a steady state infusion, again resulting in the same total propofol delivery.

was changed to a maximum of 2 μg/mL compared with a maximum of 6 μg/mL in **Fig. 2**) shows an example of procedural titration for colonoscopy. A loading dose is delivered; the scope is inserted before reaching the maximum effect; the maximum effect is reached and maintained during the most noxious part of the procedure, looping during the variable anatomy of the sigmoid colon.[4] Once the cecum has been reached, the rapid offset can be leveraged and the dose rate can be reduced or stopped, as in the example later. The effect site concentration rapidly decreases, so that when the scope is removed, patients are recovering, avoiding potential over-sedation in the recovery room.

Propofol is not the only drug that can be titrated; there are others, such as dexmedetomidine, that have a PK profile allowing for titration/infusion.[5] However, studies have shown its side effects, hemodynamic instability, and prolonged recovery limit its utility for procedural sedation.[6] As in all cases, a medications pros and cons must be considered for both patients and the procedure.

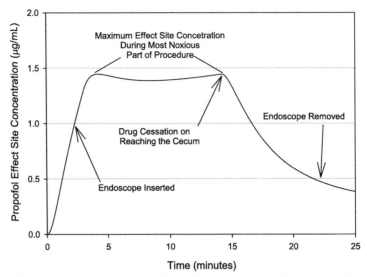

Fig. 3. A theoretic example of titration for a colonoscopy. A loading dose is delivered, and during the loading dose the endoscope is inserted. The theoretic effect site concentration is at its maximum during the most noxious part of the procedure. Once the cecum is reached, the drug is stopped, resulting in a rapid decrease in the effect site concentration. Once the endoscope is removed, the patient's effect site concentration is low, resulting in a rapid recovery.

Therefore, an ideal agent for computer- or patient-controlled sedation (PCS) would then be one whereby

- The medication titrated via a loading dose over several minutes can achieve the desired level of sedation.
- Increases can be done with incremental loading doses over a reasonable period of time.
- The infusion rate can be rapidly reduced, which will result in rapid patient recovery.
- There is a low side effect profile with hemodynamic stability.

PATIENT MONITORING AND OXYGEN DELIVERY FOR COMPUTER- OR PATIENT-CONTROLLED SEDATION
Physiologic Monitoring

A computer-controlled system especially needs to assess patients' physiology to some degree if it is going to also assess safety and not just effectiveness, which the bispectral index (BIS) and the automated responsiveness monitor provide.

The American Society of Anesthesiology (ASA) has provided guidance on what physiologic monitors should be used for sedation by a nonanesthesiologist as well as standards for basic anesthesia monitoring.[7,8] In general, the requirements are blood oxygenation, respiration, blood pressure, heart rate, and level of sedation. If deep sedation is the targeted level of sedation, then exhaled carbon dioxide and electrocardiogram (ECG) should also be included.

When looking at the cascade of injury for sedation, it is important to monitor as far upstream in the cascade as possible. **Fig. 4** shows the most common cascade of injury. An increase in drug delivery and/or a decrease in patient stimulus can result in

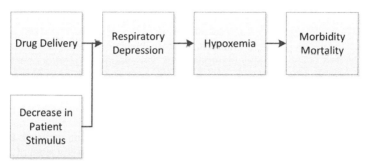

Fig. 4. The most common injury from sedation during endoscopy is low oxygenation (hypoxemia), which resulted from respiratory depression. The respiratory depression is ultimately a result of an increase in the drug delivery and/or a decrease in the patient stimulus, such as removal of the endoscope.

oversedation. Oversedation can result in respiratory depression, when the results in hypoxemia, which if profound, can result in morbidity/mortality. In assessing the level of sedation, a transition to general anesthesia determined by nonresponsive to a trapezius squeeze is not necessarily a transition to a surgical plane of general anesthesia.[9]

Clearly, per the ASA, monitoring of the level of sedation should be continually assessed. This element is the first in the cascade of injury, and the best monitor is the one that is located furthest from the injury.

As respiratory depression is next in the cascade, even for moderate sedation, it should be continually assessed, such as a precordial stethoscope or capnometer. After respiratory depression, hypoxemia should be monitored, typically via pulse oximetry.

If the drug is being titrated, the clinical team has the benefit to stop or reduce the medication, stopping the injury cascade of oversedation, apnea, hypoxemia, bradycardia/hypotension, and then morbidity/mortality.

Electroencephalogram Monitoring

Electroencephalogram (EEG) monitoring, predominately BIS being the focus of study, provides the ability to assess the effect of an anesthetic agent on the central nervous system. Controlled infusion of intravenous (IV) anesthetic agents based on the BIS provides the potential for a more controlled steady state infusion to a patient.[10] BIS has been shown to be useful in predicting recovery time and the depth of sedation of patients; however, it has not been useful in ultimately predicting patient and endoscopist satisfaction.[11–13] For this reason, it has not received widespread adoption for endoscopic sedation. In regard to use in a computer-controlled system, BIS presents unique problems. For example, at lighter levels of anesthesia (minimal/moderate sedation), even stimuli such as noise has an impact on the BIS, making the signal to noise ratio of the BIS value difficult to use in a closed loop system.[14] However, at deep levels of sedation and anesthesia, the BIS value is not impacted by these mild external stimuli.

An Automated Responsiveness Monitor

A novel automated responsiveness monitor was developed for the SEDASYS System (Ethicon Endo-Surgery, Inc, Cincinnati OH) that uses audible prompts and tactile stimulus to assess if patients are in minimal to moderate sedation.[15] This monitor is unique in that it is designed to assess sedation in a narrow range, balancing accuracy and the range of patient assessment. The monitor in the study by Doufas and colleagues[15] shows the patient is responsive in all situations before transition to deep sedation. This system provides increased accuracy for minimally to moderately sedated patients but limited utility for patients targeted for deep sedation/general anesthesia.

Ocular Microtremor Monitor

Ocular microtremor (OMT) is a novel monitoring technology that looks at the microtremors in the eye and, through assessment of those tremors, is able to assess the degree of sedation/anesthesia. OMT has been shown to correlate well with BIS, indicating a potential that this may be another means of assessing the level of neuronal activity of patients.[16] Its usefulness has yet to be proven in endoscopy and whether it will have the same shortcomings as BIS or will provide a more precise means of patient monitoring.

Oxygen Delivery

Oxygen delivery is critical in safely managing patients during sedation. By preoxygenating patients, you increase patients' partial pressure of oxygen, allowing more time during respiratory depression to manage patients' airway before they are desaturated.[17] **Fig. 5** shows an oxyhemoglobin dissociation curve with 3 slope areas highlighted. The slope when the Pao_2 is greater than 10 kPa is at its most shallow. At this point on the curve, an apneic episode will result in little if any change in the patient's oxygen saturation of arterial blood (SaO_2). If the apnea event were to continue, the patient becomes increasingly more susceptible to apnea episodes. As an apneic episode may not be total airway obstruction but shallow breathing, it is recommended

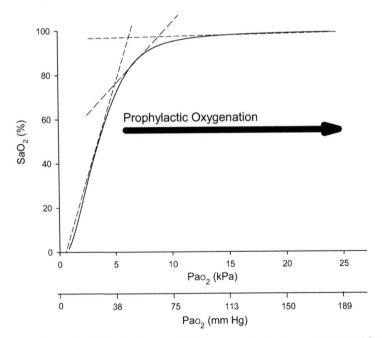

Fig. 5. An oxyhemoglobin dissociation curve is shown, constructed from an empirical fit of Pao_2 and oxygen saturation of arterial blood (SaO_2) as described by Kelman[45] and Severinghaus.[46] Three different straight lines have been drawn on the curve, indicating 3 unique slope regions.

to increase the level of oxygen delivery as patients decrease in saturation, again in a prophylactic manner. Ideally a computer-controlled sedation system should also provide a degree of automated oxygen delivery, increasing it in response to patients' oxygen saturation.

COMPUTER-CONTROLLED SEDATION SYSTEMS
Computer-Assisted Personalized Sedation

Computer-assisted personalized sedation (CAPS) systems integrate patient monitoring with oxygen and sedative delivery, enabling the administration of sedation personalized to the needs of each patient. CAPS is not target-controlled infusion (TCI), although a CAPS system can include a TCI algorithm. CAPS is not PCS, although patient feedback can be incorporated into a CAPS system. And CAPS is not closed loop, as it assists the user in the administration of sedation rather than replaces the user. These alternative means of administering sedation are discussed later in this article.[7,18]

The SEDASYS System is an example of a CAPS system. The SEDASYS System incorporates patient monitoring adhering to the ASA's guidelines for safe sedation by nonanesthesiologists[7] and a peristaltic infusion pump for the administration of propofol consistent with the dosing guidelines in the propofol package insert.[19] There are 2 components of the system, shown in **Fig. 6**.

The bedside monitoring unit (BMU) is mounted to patients' IV pole and remains with patients. The BMU monitors include pulse oximetry, ECG, and noninvasive blood pressure as shown in **Fig. 6**. It provides baseline monitoring in the preprocedure location, control and monitoring in the procedure room, and recovery monitoring in the postprocedure location. In the procedure room, the BMU is connected to the

The SEDASYS   System User Interface

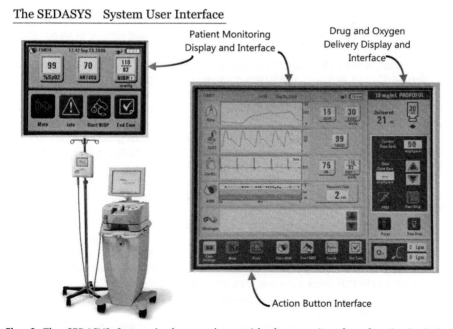

Fig. 6. The SEDASYS System is shown, along with the user interface for the bedside monitoring unit (*top left*) and the procedure room unit (*right*). (*Courtesy of* Ethicon US, LLC, Cincinnati, OH; with permission.)

procedure room unit (PRU). The PRU adds capnometry and an automated responsiveness monitor that monitors the patients' ability to respond to mild verbal and tactile stimuli. The PRU shows all physiologic monitoring, drug delivery, and oxygen delivery, as shown in **Fig. 6**. The PRU provides responsive oxygen delivery and integrates propofol delivery with the patient monitors.

This integration includes dosing limits and lockout timers and alarms that reduce or stop propofol delivery on detection of clinical signs of oversedation. The dosing limits are designed to ensure titration while maintaining minimal to moderate sedation. The limits include a maximum selection of the initial infusion rate, restriction on infusion rate increases, and a mandatory 3-minute loading dose for all infusion increases. The SEDASYS System alarms include audible and visual elements based on the patients' physiology and status of the monitors. Should patients experience hypoxemia or hypoventilation, the system will stop the propofol infusion. The system also manages oxygen delivery to patients. Oxygen is increased automatically based on the patients' peripheral oxygen saturation in a prophylactic manner, increasing at conservative thresholds.

To initiate sedation, the user selects an infusion rate to achieve a desired level of sedation. The SEDASYS System automatically calculates a loading dose and administers that dose over 3 minutes, to rapidly achieve the desired level of sedation. The user can then titrate propofol delivery, through increasing/decreasing the infusion rate or delivering a small fixed dose to treat transient discomfort, to personalize sedation to their needs throughout each portion of the endoscopic procedure.

In a 1000-patient, multicenter, randomized clinical study, the SEDASYS System was compared with sedation with benzodiazepines and opioid during routine colonoscopy and EGD.[20] A total of 496 subjects received propofol sedation with the SEDASYS System and 504 subjects received sedation using midazolam and either fentanyl or meperidine. Inclusion criteria included 18 years of age or older, body mass index less than 35, and ASA physical status I to III; exclusion criteria included allergy to any study medication, pregnancy or lactating, and diagnosed history of sleep apnea or gastroparesis.

The primary end point of this study was the area-under-the-curve of oxygen desaturation (AUC_{Desat}). AUC_{Desat} is a safety measure that integrates the incidence, depth, and duration of oxygen desaturation events.[19] The mean AUC_{Desat} for patients in the SEDASYS System group was lower (31 seconds · %) compared with patients sedated with benzodiazepines and opioids (82 seconds · %; $P = .028$).[20] Looking at a more traditional measure, fewer patients in the SEDASYS System group had an oxygen desaturation (38) compared with patients sedated with benzodiazepines and opioids (83, $P<.001$).[20]

The secondary study end points included physician satisfaction, measured by the Clinician Satisfaction with Sedation Index and patient satisfaction, measured by the Patient Satisfaction with Sedation Index (PSSI).[21]

The physicians in the study were significantly more satisfied with the administration of sedation with the SEDASYS System (PSSI = 92, 0–100 scale) compared with sedation with midazolam and fentanyl/meperidine (PSSI = 76, $P<.001$). Patients in both treatment groups were very satisfied with the sedation they received; the mean PSSI scores in both groups were approximately 90 (0–100 scale).[20] The mean amount of propofol delivered was 106 mg for colonoscopy and 70 mg for EGD, indicating minimal to moderate sedation.

The SEDASYS System is currently being used in several institutions in the United States. The clinical utility of the system, in a nonstudy application, is being assessed; further published data should be forthcoming.

Target-Controlled Infusion

Another evolving technology currently used in 96 countries (but not yet commercially available in the United States) is TCI, a technology more than 20 years old and studied in almost 600 peer-reviewed publications.[2] This delivery system administers IV agents via an infusion pump programmed to calculate and maintain the necessary infusion rate based on the PK model of a specific drug. The current TCI systems are known as open-loop systems because they operate using only a computer prediction of expected plasma concentration based on the drug profile. Unlike the other methods of computer-controlled delivery, there is traditionally no real-time feedback from patients as to the actual effects of the drug concentration.

TCI has been assessed for endoscopy in many settings. One such study was comparing propofol delivered via TCI with intermittent boluses of midazolam, alfentanil, and propofol until patients were nonresponsive to verbal commands.[22] The nadir systolic blood pressure was lower in the bolus group, as was increased hypotension for colonoscopy and bradycardia during EGD. Deeper levels of sedation were targeted when compared with CAPS discussed earlier, as reflected in the total doses of 114 ± 34 mg for EGD and 212 ± 84 mg for colonoscopy in the TCI-with-propofol group.

A question arises on whether TCI is safer or more effective than other means of sedation. One of the few randomized controlled trials done on this topic evaluated this question on patients undergoing endoscopy.[23] The first group received propofol delivered by an endoscopist. This group received an initial infusion of 30 to 50 mg of propofol followed by doses at the discretion of the endoscopist via a preprogrammed pump. The second group received deep sedation from an anesthesia provider (anesthesiologist or Certified Registered Nurse Anesthetist). The endoscopist group clearly targeted a level of sedation that was minimal to moderate with a total dose of 94 mg (similar to the dosing in the SEDASYS System study) compared with the anesthesia group that had a total dose of 260 mg. The study showed that, even with the significantly lower dose, patient satisfaction was higher in the endoscopist group. The endoscopist group also experienced fewer side effects. It is important to remember this study was first limited to 90 patients (ASA I/II) and conducted in France, so these results may very well not translate to the United States.

TCI does not always bring a benefit to the patients or physician. One study assessed the difference between traditional anesthesia delivery via propofol bolus compared with a group that received propofol using TCI.[24] Both methods allowed for control of the level of sedation; however the TCI group was associated with an increased recovery time and an increase in hypotension.

A refinement of the TCI system is a closed-loop administration method, which incorporates feedback from real-time measures of sedation, such as muscle relaxation into the computer-controlled algorithm for drug delivery. When using propofol, a closed-loop system has the potential advantage over an open-loop system of being able to provide a more precise level of sedation with a lower concentration of the drug.[25,26]

Systems in Development

There are new systems in development or in various stages of testing. The Food and Drug Administration (FDA) has not yet approved these systems; data for these systems undergoing endoscopic procedures are absent, but there is potential that they may be useful in the future.

A novel system called McSleepy (McGill University Health Centre, Canada) was developed to create a closed-loop anesthesia system, involving the use of BIS, analgoscore, and phonomyography as the control variables, delivering pharmacologic agents for analgesia, hypnosis, and neuromuscular blockade.[27] The system included a touch screen to provide an interface for bidirectional communication regarding the stage of anesthesia and prompts to the anesthesiologist regarding required actions, such as bag mask ventilation or intubation. In general, the system was found to provide clinical usefulness to the anesthesiologist in regard to precise drug control. The FDA has not approved this system for use.

Another device, currently under investigation, called iControl-RP (Fraser Health, BC), is different in that it is a closed-loop system, using EEG data to control a propofol and remifentanil, with an estimated completion date of February 2016.[28] Currently the study is looking at surgical procedures; but it is reasonable to assume this and other technologies will continue to advance, allowing for closed-loop control of sedation at some point in the future. The FDA has not approved this system for use.

PATIENT-CONTROLLED INFUSION SYSTEMS

Patient-controlled analgesia (PCA) is not a new concept and has been around since the early 1960 to 1970s, originally used to assist in the management of noxious stimulus, such as postoperative pain and labor.[29,30] PCS more recently has been introduced, which has built on PCA. PCS allows patients to have some control over the delivery of sedatives and/or analgesics via a computerized pump. Typically the patient control is a handheld button, which, when activated by patients, provides either a bolus or increase to the medication delivered during procedures that have noxious stimulus.[31] The pump administers predetermined boluses of IV medication typically against a continuous background infusion. The intent of these systems is to provide a means whereby patients can manage the degree of sedation based on their level of discomfort while maintaining a level of sedation not greater than what is needed by patients.

PCS has been studied for endoscopy procedures showing both safety and effectiveness in many studies.[32–41] Most of these studies were done outside of the United States; in general, PCS has not gained widespread adoption for endoscopy within the United States. These studies using PCS looked at different medications, including propofol, dexmedetomidine (both IV and intranasal), alfentanil, inhaled methoxyflurane, as well as others in an attempt to provide safe and effective sedation with a high degree of patient satisfaction. In general, patient recovery is faster because less total medication is used than with conventional sedation methods. PCS may not be suitable for patients who do not have the willingness or capacity to comply with instructions.

Mazanikov and his colleagues[32] from Helsinki, Finland have extensively studied PCS. In one study they compared propofol delivered via TCI and PCS during an endoscopic retrograde cholangiopancreatography (ECRP). What they found was that there was no statistical difference between these two approaches in terms of safety and satisfaction. Propofol consumption was less for the PCS group, and patients were at a comparable level of sedation in the recovery room. This finding led the investigators to provide PCS as a viable option compared with TCI, as PCS is simpler to administer, has a similar (or potentially improved) safety profile, and has a reduced consumption of sedative.

It has also been shown that PCS using propofol/alfentanil has the potential to provide a safer sedation experience when compared with midazolam/meperidine while providing increased patient satisfaction along with a shorter recovery.[40] PCS has also been compared with anesthetist-delivered sedation. In a double-blinded study, patients either managed their sedation using PCS with propofol or an anesthesiologist delivered the propofol.[42] The study found that patient and endoscopist satisfaction were similar for both groups; PCS patients were sedated more slowly; and the level of sedation was not as deep compared with the anesthesiologist. The anesthesiologist group had an increased number of hypotensive episodes. There was no difference in procedural recall or recovery times.

However, PCS has been found to have differing results in regard to satisfaction.[43] Studies have shown a decrease in satisfaction, equivalent satisfaction, and greater satisfaction compared with non–patient-controlled satisfaction.[34,39,44] Given these data, it is difficult to assess if PCS provides clinical benefits compared with physician-directed sedation.

Clearly part of the success or failure in the use of PCS is the proper selection of medications. As referenced earlier, dexmedetomidine has been shown to be less than ideal given its side effects, hemodynamic instability, and prolonged recovery.[6] In a study of alcoholic patients receiving an ERCP comparing dexmedetomidine with placebo with PCS (propofol/alfentanil) available as a means of rescue medication, all patients who received dexmedetomidine required additional sedation using propofol/alfentanil delivered via PCS.[33] Interestingly, a study looking at intranasal dexmedetomidine delivered for EGD procedures, followed by PCS with propofol/alfentanil, demonstrated a significant decrease in the use of propofol/alfentanil, indicating the route of administration and synergies between medications is as critical as medication selection.[35] Although these referenced studies all reference alfentanil as the opioid, remifentanil has also been shown to be as effective for endoscopic procedures.[39,41]

PCS is not limited to the use of propofol. For instance, one study done in Israel looked at supplementing a midazolam/meperidine regimen with a pump that supported additional doses of meperidine under the control of patients.[37] In this case they showed that this method of administration (supplemental meperidine doses only using PCS) was as safe and effective as their traditional means of sedation.

Other novel agents, in regard to endoscopy, may be used for PCS. A study compared inhaled methoxyflurane via PCS with traditional midazolam/fentanyl for colonoscopy.[38] The study found that PCS with methoxyflurane was not associated with desaturation, had faster recovery times, and did not impact procedural success and polyp detection. Eight percent of the PCS patients did require additional IV midazolam/fentanyl, so, although not a total replacement, the study population did see significant benefits.

Clearly PCS has a potential to provide sedation for endoscopic procedures, either in combination with a traditional drug delivery as a supplement or as a standalone method. More work in the United States needs to be done before having an on-label means of using PCS for certain medications, such as propofol and remifentanil. Given existing regulatory and safety concerns from many parties, it is unlikely PCS will provide an on-label solution to US delivery of propofol in the near future.

SUMMARY

Endoscopic sedation has continued to evolve, increasing patients' comfort while improving patients' safety. This has required investigating multiple approaches, including computer- or PCS. The emerging technologies discussed are demonstrating optimization through the titration of drug delivery, targeting lighter levels of sedation, adequate patient monitoring, cessation, or reduction of drug delivery based on patient assessment, with prophylactic oxygenation providing safe and effective sedation. Computer- or patient-controlled systems provide the possibility to advance sedation as a science and standardize administration and monitoring parameters to gastroen-terologists and anesthesia providers alike. These technologies present paradigm shifts in the current use of bolus administration that will require and perhaps allow training standardization as well. The cost-effectiveness of these platforms is beyond the scope of this discussion, and further studies are needed to determine the role of these technologies in endoscopic sedation.

REFERENCES

1. Green SM. Research advances in procedural sedation and analgesia. Ann Emerg Med 2007;49(1):31–6.
2. Absalom AR, Glen JI, Zwart GJC, et al. Target-controlled infusion. Anesth Analg 2015;122(1):1.
3. Rudkin GE, Osborne GA, Finn BP, et al. Intra-operative patient-controlled seda-tion. Anaesthesia 1992;47(5):376–81.
4. Shah SG, Brooker JC, Thapar C, et al. Patient pain during colonoscopy: an analysis using real-time magnetic endoscope imaging. Endoscopy 2002;34(6):435–40.
5. Dyck JB, Maze M, Haack C, et al. Computer-controlled infusion of intravenous dexmedetomidine hydrochloride in adult human volunteers. Anesthesiology 1993;78(5):821–8.
6. Jalowiecki P, Rudner R, Gonciarz M, et al. Sole use of dexmedetomidine has limited utility for conscious sedation during outpatient colonoscopy. Anesthesi-ology 2005;103(2):269–73.
7. American Society of Anesthesiologists Task Force on Sedation and Analgesia by Non-Anesthesiologists. Practice guidelines for sedation and analgesia by non-anesthesiologists. Anesthesiology 2002;96(4):1004–17.
8. Approved by the ASA House of Delegates on October 21, 1986 last amended on, October 20, 2010, and last affirmed on October 28 2015. Standards for Basic Anesthetic Monitoring. Available at: http://www.asahq.org/.../standards-for-basic-anesthetic-monitoring/en/1.
9. Kim TK, Niklewski PJ, Martin JF, et al. Enhancing a sedation score to include truly noxious stimulation: the Extended Observer's Assessment of Alertness and Seda-tion (EOAA/S). Br J Anaesth 2015;115(4):569–77.
10. Liu N, Hafiani EM, Le Guen M. Closed-loop anesthesia based on neuromonitor-ing. In: Ehrenfeld JM, Cannesson M, editors. Monitoring technologies in acute care environments. Springer; 2014. p. 109–15.
11. Mitty RD, Moses PL, Pleskow DK. BIS monitoring predicts recovery time in patients receiving intraprocedural midazolam during endoscopy. Gastrointest Endosc 2004;59(5):P129.
12. Patel S, Vargo J, Trolli P, et al. Correlation of patient satisfaction to sedation levels detected by bispectral index (BIS) using moderate sedation (MS). Gastrointest Endosc 2004;59(5):P129.
13. Cohen LB, Manzi DJ, Moses PL, et al. Bispectral index (BIS) correlates well with American Society for Anesthesiology (ASA) sedation levels during colonoscopy performed with propofol sedation. Gastrointest Endosc 2005;61(5):AB112.
14. Kim DW, Kil HY, White PF. The effect of noise on the bispectral index during pro-pofol sedation. Anesth Analg 2001;93(5):1170–3.
15. Doufas AG, Morioka N, Mahgoub AN, et al. Automated responsiveness monitor to titrate propofol sedation. Anesth Analg 2009;109(3):778.
16. Kevin LG. Comparison of ocular microtremor and bispectral index during sevo-flurane anaesthesiadagger. Br J Anaesth 2002;89(4):551–5.

17. Weingart SD, Levitan RM. Preoxygenation and prevention of desaturation during emergency airway management. Ann Emerg Med 2012;59(3):165–75.e1.
18. Niklewski PJ, Phero JC, Martin JF, et al. A novel index of hypoxemia for assessment of risk during procedural sedation. Anesth Analg 2014;119(4):848–56.
19. AstraZeneca. Diprivan (propofol) injectable emulsion. Techniques. AstraZeneca Pharmaceuticals; 2005. p. 1–4.
20. Pambianco DJ, Vargo JJ, Pruitt RE, et al. Computer-assisted personalized sedation for upper endoscopy and colonoscopy: a comparative, multicenter randomized study. Gastrointest Endosc 2011;73(4):765–72.
21. Vargo J, Howard K, Petrillo J, et al. Development and validation of the patient and clinician sedation satisfaction index for colonoscopy and upper endoscopy. Clin Gastroenterol Hepatol 2009;7(2):156–62.
22. Chan W-H, Chang S-L, Lin C-S, et al. Target-controlled infusion of propofol versus intermittent bolus of a sedative cocktail regimen in deep sedation for gastrointestinal endoscopy: comparison of cardiovascular and respiratory parameters. J Dig Dis 2014;15(1):18–26.
23. Poincloux L, Laquière A, Bazin J-E, et al. A randomized controlled trial of endoscopist vs. anaesthetist-administered sedation for colonoscopy. Dig Liver Dis 2011;43(7):553–8.
24. Riphaus A, Geist C. Intermittent manually controlled versus continuous infusion of propofol for deep sedation during interventional endoscopy: a prospective randomized trial. Scand J Gastroenterol 2012;47(8–9):1078–85.
25. Fanti L, Gemma M, Agostoni M, et al. Target controlled infusion for non-anaesthesiologist propofol sedation during gastrointestinal endoscopy: the first double blind randomized controlled trial. Dig Liver Dis 2015;47(7):566–71.
26. Leslie K, Absalom A, Kenny GNC. Closed loop control of sedation for colonoscopy using the bispectral index. Anaesthesia 2002;57(7):693–7.
27. Wehbe M, Arbeid E, Cyr S, et al. A technical description of a novel pharmacological anesthesia robot. J Clin Monit Comput 2014;28(1):27–34.
28. ClinicalTrials.Gov. Closed-loop control of anesthesia: controlled delivery of remifentanil and propofol - full text view - ClinicalTrials.gov. Available at: https://clinicaltrials.gov/ct2/show/NCT01771263. Accessed January 11, 2016.
29. Yakaitis RW, Cooke JE, Redding JS. Self-administered methoxyflurane for postoperative pain: effectiveness and patient acceptance. Anesth Analg 1972; 51(2):208–12.
30. Scott JS. Obstetric analgesia. A consideration of labor pain and a patient-controlled technique for its relief with meperidine. Am J Obstet Gynecol 1970; 106(7):959–78.
31. Atkins JH, Mandel JE. Recent advances in patient-controlled sedation. Curr Opin Anaesthesiol 2008;21(6):759–65.
32. Mazanikov M, Udd M, Kylänpää L, et al. A randomized comparison of target-controlled propofol infusion and patient-controlled sedation during ERCP. Endoscopy 2013;45(11):915–9.
33. Mazanikov M, Udd M, Kylänpää L, et al. Dexmedetomidine impairs success of patient-controlled sedation in alcoholics during ERCP: a randomized, double-blind, placebo-controlled study. Surg Endosc 2013;27(6):2163–8.
34. Maurice-Szamburski A, Loundou A, Auquier P, et al. Effect of patient-controlled sedation with propofol on patient satisfaction: a randomized study. Ann Fr Anesth Reanim 2013;32(12):e171–5.

35. Cheung CW, Qiu Q, Liu J, et al. Intranasal dexmedetomidine in combination with patient-controlled sedation during upper gastrointestinal endoscopy: a randomised trial. Acta Anaesthesiol Scand 2015;59(2):215–23.
36. Liu SYW, Poon CM, Leung TL, et al. Nurse-administered propofol-alfentanil sedation using a patient-controlled analgesia pump compared with opioid-benzodiazepine sedation for outpatient colonoscopy. Endoscopy 2009;41(6):522–8.
37. Stermer E, Gaitini L, Yudashkin M, et al. Patient-controlled analgesia for conscious sedation during colonoscopy: a randomized controlled study. Gastrointest Endosc 2000;51(3):278–81.
38. Nguyen NQ, Toscano L, Lawrence M, et al. Patient-controlled analgesia with inhaled methoxyflurane versus conventional endoscopist-provided sedation for colonoscopy: a randomized multicenter trial. Gastrointest Endosc 2013;78(6): 892–901.
39. Mazanikov M, Udd M, Kylänpää L, et al. Patient-controlled sedation with propofol and remifentanil for ERCP: a randomized, controlled study. Gastrointest Endosc 2011;73(2):260–6.
40. Külling D, Fantin AC, Biro P, et al. Safer colonoscopy with patient-controlled analgesia and sedation with propofol and alfentanil. Gastrointest Endosc 2001; 54(1):1–7.
41. Fanti L, Agostoni M, Gemma M, et al. Two dosages of remifentanil for patient-controlled analgesia vs. meperidine during colonoscopy: a prospective randomized controlled trial. Dig Liver Dis 2013;45(4):310–5.
42. Stonell CA, Leslie K, Absalom AR. Effect-site targeted patient-controlled sedation with propofol: comparison with anaesthetist administration for colonoscopy. Anaesthesia 2006;61(3):240–7.
43. Sheahan CG, Mathews DM. Monitoring and delivery of sedation. Br J Anaesth 2014;113(Suppl):ii37–47.
44. Ng JM, Kong CF, Nyam D. Patient-controlled sedation with propofol for colonoscopy. Gastrointest Endosc 2001;54(1):8–13.
45. Kelman GR. Digital computer subroutine for the conversion of oxygen tension into saturation. J Appl Physiol 1966;21(4):1375–6.
46. Severinghaus JW. Simple, accurate equations for human blood O2 dissociation computations. J Appl Physiol 1979;46(3):599–602.

On the Horizon
The Future of Procedural Sedation

 CrossMark

Gursimran S. Kochhar, MD[a], Anant Gill, MBBS[b], John J. Vargo, MD, MPH[c],*

KEYWORDS

- Sedation • Propofol • Endoscopic sedation

KEY POINTS

- Endoscopic sedation has evolved substantially over the past decade.
- Patient safety and comfort remain the center of focus.
- Even though a formal curriculum has been developed, there has not been, to the authors' knowledge, a competency-based sedation training program that has been implemented for endoscopic procedural sedation.

INTRODUCTION

According to the standards of practice committee of the American Society for Gastrointestinal Endoscopy (ASGE), "sedation is defined as a drug-induced depression in level of consciousness."[1] Sedation is a fundamental aspect of gastrointestinal endoscopy (GIE) because it reduces anxiety and patient discomfort and also allows for better examination during endoscopy, thereby improving patient outcomes. The goal of sedation is to achieve a balance between the comfort aspects while preserving patient safety. Although sedation improves a patient's tolerance, it also increases both the cost and the risks of complications. Sedation itself is responsible for about 50% of all GIE complications.[2,3] Sedation can be divided into 4 levels, ranging from minimal sedation to moderate, deep, and general anesthesia. Differences between various stages of sedation are described in **Table 1**. The most commonly used form of sedation in GIE is moderate sedation, also known as "conscious sedation." Some of the most commonly used agents for sedation and their antagonists in GIE are listed in **Boxes 1** and **2**, respectively. The targeted level of sedation depends on various factors like the type of examination, patient comorbidities, and the American Society of

Conflict of Interest: The authors declared no financial conflict of interest pertaining to this article.
[a] Department of Gastroenterology and Hepatology, Digestive Disease Institute, Cleveland Clinic, Cleveland, OH, USA; [b] Saraswathi Institute of Medical Sciences, Anwarpur, Uttar Pradesh, India; [c] Department of Gastroenterology and Hepatology, Digestive Disease Institute, Cleveland Clinic, Cleveland Clinic Foundation, A-30, 9500 Euclid Avenue, Cleveland, OH, USA
* Corresponding author.
E-mail address: vargoj@ccf.org

Table 1 Levels of sedation and anesthesia				
	Minimal Sedation	**Moderate Sedation**	**Deep Sedation**	**General Anesthesia**
Responsiveness	Normal response to verbal stimulation	Purposeful response to verbal or tactile stimulation	Purposeful response after repeated or painful stimulation	Unarousable even with painful stimulus
Airway	Unaffected	No intervention required	Intervention may be required	Intervention often required
Spontaneous ventilation	Unaffected	Adequate	May be inadequate	Frequently inadequate
Cardiovascular function	Unaffected	Usually maintained	Usually maintained	May be impaired

From Standards of Practice Committee of the American Society for Gastrointestinal Endoscopy, Lichtenstein DR, Jagannath S, et al. Sedation and anesthesia in GI endoscopy. Gastrointest Endosc 2008;68:815–26; with permission.

Anesthesiology (ASA) disease classification (**Table 2**). Although the gastroenterology community is well versed in traditional sedation methods, the authors would like to put forth recent advances in endoscopic sedation, newer anesthesia medications, or combination methods that might be of use in the future of GIE, current aspects of sedation training available, and quality assessment of sedation during GIE.

TRAINING IN SEDATION FOR ENDOSCOPY

Given the recent advances in GIE sedation, training forms the cornerstone of successful sedation practices for the current and future gastroenterologist. The Multisociety Sedation Curriculum for Gastrointestinal Endoscopy (MSCGE) outlines a detailed, systemic approach for sedation describing pharmacology, informed consent, periprocedural assessment, levels of sedation, and anesthesiologist assistance for endoscopic procedure.[4] This curriculum is beneficial for both the training individual and the practicing gastroenterologist to boost their knowledge and skills. The American Association for the Study of Liver Diseases, the American College of Gastroenterology, the American Gastroenterological Association, Society for "Gastroenterology

Box 1 Most commonly used agents in sedation in gastrointestinal endoscopy
1. Dexmedetomidine
2. Diazepam
3. Diphenhydramine
4. Droperidol
5. Fentanyl
6. Meperidine
7. Midazolam
8. Propofol

Box 2
Commonly used antagonist medication in sedation in gastrointestinal endoscopy

Naloxone: Fentanyl, Meperidine

Flumazenil: Diazepam, Midazolam

Nurse and Associates", and the ASGE all contributed to this MSCGE. Representatives from these societies helped in forming this curriculum, keeping in mind the utmost importance of research based on ethics, humanism, and professionalism.

The endoscopist must have a complete understanding of sedation agents, including pharmacokinetics and pharmacodynamics, adverse effects, and drug interactions.[4] As the main focus is the comfort and safety of the patient during the procedure, the patient's detailed medical history, medications, intubation assessment, anxiety, and pain intolerance should be reviewed. Benzodiazepines and opioids were previously commonly used agents, but, with time, newer sedation agents have been used. In most cases, moderate sedation is used, but a trainee should be knowledgeable in titrating the agents to produce the required level of sedation.[4]

Informed consent for endoscopic sedation is an obligation for the physician, from both ethical and legal standpoints. A trainee should be well versed with the process of informed consent. Periprocedure assessment is another important part of

Table 2
American Society of Anesthesiology physical status classification

PS1	Normal healthy patient	No organic, physiologic, or psychiatric disturbance; excludes the very young and very old; healthy with good exercise tolerance
PS2	Patients with mild systemic disease	No functional limitations; has well controlled disease of 1 body system; controlled hypertension or diabetes without systemic side effects; cigarette smoking without COPD; mild obesity; pregnancy
PS3	Patients with severe systemic disease	Some functional limitation; has controlled disease of >1 body system or 1 major system; no immediate danger of death; controlled CHF, stable angina, previous heart attack, poorly controlled hypertension, morbid obesity, chronic renal failure, bronchospastic disease with intermittent symptoms
PS4	Patients with severe systemic disease that is constant threat to life	Has at least 1 severe disease that is poorly controlled or at end stage; possible risk of death; unstable angina, symptomatic COPD, symptomatic CHF, hepatorenal failure
PS5	Moribound patients who are not expected to survive without operation	Not expected to survive >24 h without surgery; imminent risk of death; multiorgan failure, sepsis syndrome with hemodynamic instability, hypothermia, poorly controlled coagulopathy
PS6	A declared brain-dead patient whose organs are being removed for donor purposes	—

Abbreviations: CHF, congestive heart failure; COPD, chronic obstructive pulmonary disease; PS, physical status.

endoscopic sedation, which includes the medical and sedation history of the patient while keeping the risks of sedation in mind. Before the procedure, a trainee should be able to assess the patient according to the ASA physical status classification (see **Table 2**). The patient's airway should be evaluated, which covers the structure of the neck, hyoid mental distance, cervical spine, and oropharynx. The trainee should understand the anatomy of the oral cavity, which facilitates endotracheal intubation, and keep in mind the modified Mallampati classification, which has 4 grades (grade 1 means a complete visibility of the soft palate, uvula, and tonsils, and grade 4 means only the hard palate is visible). The trainee should be able to recognize whether anesthesiologist assistance is required for the procedure that needs general anesthesia or deep sedation. The trainee must be facile with intraprocedure and postprocedure assessment, including physiologic parameters and levels of sedation.

The trainee should be well prepared to rescue the patient in the event of a deeper sedation than what was targeted. Usually, opioids and benzodiazepines are used to achieve moderate sedation, but propofol can be used with other agents for moderate sedation and alone for deep sedation. An endoscopist should precisely identify arrhythmias and take proper measures to manage them. A trainee should have an Advanced Cardiac Life Support (ACLS) certificate or have had training in an Advanced Trauma Life Support course and should have experience in airway training; the indications for the use of naloxone and flumazenil are also required.[4]

Postprocedure assessment is a continuation of intraprocedure monitoring and evaluates the physiologic recovery of the patient. The trainee should be familiar with the Post Anesthetic Discharge Scoring System (ie, vital signs, activity, mental status, pain, nausea, vomiting, bleeding) or the Aldrete Score (ie, respiration, oxygen saturation, consciousness, circulation; **Box 3**). The patient procedure should be accompanied by an adult and should not drive.

The assessment of competency is of utmost importance in endoscopic sedation and should be tested clinically and in written examinations. Trainees should work on simulators (if available) before they start in the procedure room. Simulator-based training using a full-scale patient simulator as an adjunct to practical courses may improve the skills of trainees. MSCGE curricula recommend the use of such simulator programs. Simulation-based sedation training includes both technical and human performance aspects of managing adverse events; it also allows training in pharmacology, appropriate selection of sedative drugs for use in endoscopic procedures, pertinent monitoring techniques, and management of complications of intravenous sedation, including basic to advanced life support and recovery care. One study performed during a training course for sedation during endoscopy showed significant improvement in examination test scores of attendees at the end of 3 hours of training that included hands-on management on a full-scale patient simulator compared with those before training.[5] It provides trainees with the specified knowledge and skills during a condensed period.

According to the American Board of Internal Medicine, evaluations should be transparent and based on the trainee's medical knowledge, ACLS protocols, patient care, practice-based learning and system-based learning, interpersonal and communication skills, and feedback from nurses, patients, and technicians.

Currently published guidelines emphasize all endoscopists and endoscopy nurses using nonanesthesia provider-administered propofol (NAAP) to have the appropriate education and practical training. The ASGE recommends that training courses include theoretical and practical parts, followed by an examination and certified documentation of the training. An endoscopist using NAAP must be trained in ACLS, and nurses should, at least, be trained in basic life support.

> **Box 3**
> **Aldrete scoring system**
>
> *Respiration*
>
> 2 = Able to take deep breath and cough
>
> 1 = Dyspnea/shallow breathing
>
> 0 = Apnea
>
> *Oxygen saturation*
>
> 2 = Maintains >92% on room air
>
> 1 = Needs O_2 inhalation to maintain O_2 saturation >90%
>
> *Consciousness*
>
> 2 = Fully awake
>
> 1 = Arousable on calling
>
> 0 = Not responding
>
> *Circulation*
>
> 2 = BP ± 20 mm Hg preprocedurally
>
> 1 = BP ± 20 to 50 mm Hg preprocedurally
>
> 0 = BP ± 50 mm Hg preprocedurally
>
> *Activity*
>
> 2 = Able to move 4 extremities
>
> 1 = Able to move 2 extremities
>
> 0 = Able to move 0 extremities
>
> Total score is 10.
>
> Patient scoring ≥8 and returned to similar preoperative status are fit for transition to phase II recovery.

As of now, not many fellowship training programs have a dedicated training time that is devoted toward endoscopic sedation training. The authors think there should be a graded curriculum of teaching endoscopic sedation in fellowship programs. Training programs are encouraged to use simulator-based training to train fellows in an initial period of training, followed by training under direct supervision of a staff physician. Curriculum should be designed to move from conscious sedation to AAP to NAAP. The training program should assess competency of fellows in sedation at regular intervals during their training.

SEDATION AGENTS

Over the years, various sedation agents have been tried and used for GIE. **Box 1** presents a brief list of GIE sedation agents. Although midazolam and propofol remain the cornerstones of GIE sedation, various other newer agents are also being tested as feasible alternatives to the traditional agents. For the purpose of this review, the use of propofol is discussed in detail, and some of the newer agents are briefly touched upon.

Propofol

Propofol (2,6-diisopropylphenol) is currently the most common and popular hypnotic agent used for procedural sedation. It is an ultra-short-acting agent with sedative, amnestic, and hypnotic effects.[6] Because of these properties, anesthesiologists and gastroenterologists all over the world have been increasingly using propofol to replace classical sedation over the last decade. Propofol rapidly crosses the blood-brain barrier and causes potentiation of the γ-aminobutyric acid-A receptor in the brain.[6] It is 98% plasma protein-bound and is rapidly metabolized in the liver. Typically, the time from administration to its onset of action is 30 to 60 seconds, and its duration of effect is up to 4 to 8 minutes. It is now, essentially, the agent of choice for endoscopic sedation. In a recent nationwide US survey, 25.7% of gastroenterologist responders preferred propofol.[7] Propofol also potentiates the central nervous system effects of narcotic analgesics and sedatives such as benzodiazepines, barbiturates, and others, thereby helping reducing the dose of these medications administered.

Some of the potential side effects of propofol include pain at the injection site, which can occur in up to in 30% of patients receiving the drug.[8] It also causes a decrease in cardiac output, systemic vascular resistance, and a drop in blood pressure (BP). It also causes respiratory depression. All these effects can be reversed rapidly with a dose reduction or the interruption of infusion.[9] As of now, there is no reversal agent for propofol. Propofol comes with a package warning that agent should only be given by persons trained in the administration of general anesthesia. The ASA released a directive stating propofol "must only be used by healthcare provider with specialized training in airway management." This package warning has both medical and legal implications regarding patient safety issues. Secondary to the directive, the administration of propofol by nonanesthesiologists in the United States has waned popularity. Across the United States, propofol is now only administered by an anesthesiologist or a Certified Nurse Anesthetist who works with an anesthesiologist.

Studies have shown a higher after-procedure patient satisfaction with propofol versus conscious sedation agents for colonoscopy,[10] endoscopic ultrasound,[11] and endoscopic retrograde cholangiopancreatography (ERCP),[12] but not for esophagogastroduodenoscopy (EGD).[10] It is also known that time to sedation and recovery is also shorter with propofol versus traditional sedation. Because of the above-mentioned reasons, new evidence has emerged in recent years regarding the use of NAAP and monitored anesthesia care (MAC) for GIE.[13] NAAP refers to administration of propofol by either a gastroenterologist or a registered nurse under the supervision of the endoscopist.

A recent meta-analysis looked at the pooled results of NAAP and anesthesia provider-administered propofol (AAP) studies and reported the same rates of hypoxia and airway intervention in both arms.[14] Several other significant studies, including a worldwide safety survey of 646,080 procedures with NAAP, concluded NAAP is safe to use for GIE.[15]

Recently, a large prospective study was done in Sao Paulo, Brazil. In this prospective study, patients undergoing routine EGD and colonoscopies were enrolled in the study. Patients were divided into 2 groups: one NAAP group and another MAC group. A total of 2000 patients were enrolled in 2 groups with 1000 per group. The investigators reported that 12.8% of patients in the NAAP group experienced hypoxemia compared with 11.2% in MAC group. The investigators concluded that there were no notable differences in any outcomes between the 2 groups.[16] In another study from Australia, a retrospective chart review was done, in which a total of 33,539 NAAP procedures were identified. Complications were recorded based on medical emergency team calls during those procedures. A total of 23 calls were noted, and patients were discharged the same day with no intervention in 16 of the calls, whereas

7 calls led to endotracheal intubation, of which 2 patients died (and both patients were either ASA III or ASA IV).[17]

Based on the current mounting evidence on the safety and efficacy of NAAP, the European Society of Gastrointestinal Endoscopy and the European Society of Gastroenterology and Endoscopy Nurses and Associates released joint guidelines for the use of NAAP.[13] They recommended that, for patients undergoing NAAP, health care professionals should assess the patient's ASA classification, physical status, age, body mass index (BMI), Mallampati classification, and the risk factors for obstructive sleep apnea (OSA) before the procedure. They also indicate that any patient with an ASA class II or lower and Mallampati class less than 3 may undergo NAAP, and patients with an ASA classification at or above III or any severe comorbidity, an anesthesiologist should be involved in the procedure. They also suggest considering the use of capnography during NAAP, especially in long procedures and in patients with significant comorbidities. Regarding the administration of propofol, they recommend using intermittent bolus infusion or perfusion systems, including target-controlled infusion. Regarding the discharge of patients after NAAP, they recommend using a postanesthetic discharge scoring system (PADSS) to determine which patient can be discharged. The group also recommends that patients in ASA class II or higher should, upon discharge, be accompanied by a caregiver and refrain from driving, drinking alcohol, operating heavy machinery, or engaging in legally binding decisions for 24 hours.

Alternative Sedation Agents

Propofol has been the leader in sedation for GIE in the last decade. Given that the administration of propofol is done primarily by an anesthesiologist, the cost of the procedures involving propofol has been driven increasing. This increased cost is a driving factor to find an alternative sedative that is safe and can be administered by an endoscopist without compromising patient comfort, safety, and quality of the procedures. Various medications in different combinations have been explored, and some of them are reviewed in this article.

Dexmedetomidine

Dexmedetomidine (DEX) is a potent, selective α2-adrenoceptor agonist. Its specificity for α2-adrenoceptor is 8 times that of clonidine.[18] Its other advantages include anxiolysis and analgesia without respiratory depression. DEX use during MAC has been evaluated in few studies.[19] More recently, its safety profile has been assessed in various cardiology procedures.[20] Its use as a sole sedative agent is still not accepted, because concrete evidence in this regard is still lacking.

Remifentanil

Remifentanil is an opioid with potent analgesic properties. It has a short half-life and time-independent context-sensitive half-time.[21] Remifentanil carries a risk of respiratory depression. A group in France studied the use of remifentanil as a solo agent for sedation. The study had 91 patients, each receiving target-controlled infusion, with an initial target of 2 ng/mL. Thirty-seven percent of patients reported short-duration respiratory depression, which is a concerning finding, if the patient is in the care of practitioners untrained or unfamiliar with airway management.[22] Remifentanil, given its nonhepatic metabolic clearance, can be safely used in patients with hepatic dysfunction.[21] Few other studies have looked at the use of remifentanil in GIE. Bouvet and colleagues[23] recommended the use of remifentanil as an alternative to propofol. Also, when remifentanil was used in combination with an etomidate infusion, the combination showed a similar cardiovascular safety profile as propofol for use during colonoscopy.[24]

Ketamine

Ketamine is a phencyclidine derivative that acts on various receptors, including N-methyl-D-aspartate, dopamine 2, and noradrenalin. Ketamine also has a short half-life, and, like remifentanil, it also has a time-independent context-sensitive half-time.[21] The biggest advantage of ketamine over other sedatives (including propofol) is its ability to provide analgesia without apnea or respiratory depression. Ketamine does not cause depression of the airway reflexes.[21] There are limited data on the use of ketamine as a single agent or in combination with midazolam in GIE. It is used more commonly in the pediatric population because it causes less apnea.[25] Nevertheless, despite its lack of effects on the respiratory system, ketamine has not gained popularity because of the emergence phenomenon, especially in adults.[21] Some people advocate using midazolam in conjunction with ketamine to obliterate some of the effects of emergence.

Ketofol is a combination of ketamine and propofol that has also gained attention recently. Usually, the dose can be mixed in a 1:1 ratio or can be given sequentially.[22] There is no evidence in GIE that ketofol is better than either agent alone; it has been used with some success in the emergency department, though.[26]

Fospropofol

Fospropofol is one of the newer agents approved in 2008 by the US Food and Drug Administration. It is essentially a prodrug formulation of propofol. Because of this, it does not cause side effects like burning at the injection site, although it can cause pruritus or perineal paresthesia.[22] Investigations are ongoing to study its use in GIE. So far, published literature regarding fospropofol use in GIE has not indicated a higher risk of adverse events for fospropofol.[27,28]

Remimazolam

Remimazolam (CNS7056) is a new drug emerging in the field of sedation and anesthesia and is a combination of midazolam and remifentanil, 2 of the most well-studied drugs in GIE. It acts on the same receptors as midazolam: γ-aminobutyric acid. It has an organ-independent elimination similar to remifentanil.[22,29] So far, 4 clinical trials have evaluated remimazolam for GIE.[29] Pambianco and colleagues[29] studied the use of remimazolam versus midazolam for colonoscopies. The investigators did use fentanyl for pain relief as needed in addition to remimazolam during the procedure. The study group showed a rapid onset of action that resulted in earlier and deeper sedation when compared with midazolam. The recovery times were short and similar for both groups. Adverse events between both the groups were similar. Discharge times between both study groups did not differ.[29] More than 900 patients across 4 phase II clinical trials have been exposed to remimazolam with no additional reported safety concerns than previously expected with conscious sedation.[29] Phase III clinical trials are needed to achieve a label similar to midazolam.

SEDATION IN SPECIAL POPULATIONS UNDERGOING GASTROINTESTINAL ENDOSCOPY

With the expansion of the use of NAAP and propofol in general for GIE comes concerns of safety for patients, especially in certain patient populations like the elderly, patients with OSA, and patients with end-stage liver disease or cirrhosis.

In the elderly population, an awareness of the pharmacokinetics of the drugs administered is very important. The onset of action is slower in the elderly, and these patients are at a higher risk of cardiopulmonary complications and aspirations.[30] The recovery time is also slower in this population, so the anesthesia medications in this group should be titrated slowly. Currently, there is no direct evidence regarding the use of NAAP exclusively for elderly populations. From the existing evidence, no increase in the incidence of complications was found in this group.

OSA is an underdiagnosed medical condition, given that an estimated 82% of men and 92% of women with moderate to severe sleep apnea are undiagnosed.[31] Higher morbidity and mortality are seen in patients with OSA due to a higher risk of postoperative adverse events such as cardiac events and acute respiratory failure.[32,33] Various questionnaires are available to screen patients for OSA. The STOP-BANG questionnaire is a list of 8 questions for patients that have been designed to be easy to complete and interpret. The STOP-BANG questionnaire encompasses loud snoring, tiredness, observed apnea, high BP, high BMI, age, and neck circumference. STOP-BANG is one of the most frequently used tools to screen for OSA before endoscopy because it has high negative predictive value for moderate and severe OSA.[34] Various studies, with both NAAP and AAP, have suggested a higher risk of hypoxemia during GIE because of sedation in patients with OSA. Currently, there seems to be no evidence to suggest a higher risk of complications in patients with OSA and NAAP. Nevertheless, the authors consider in the use of AAP in patients with OSA, and especially for the patients with an ASA classification at or above III.

Another important subpopulation of patients to consider in sedation is patients with cirrhosis. Cirrhosis is a significant comorbid condition with a significant impact on patients' overall health, including cardiovascular health. Sedation with propofol has always been a concern in cirrhotic patients because propofol is mainly metabolized in the liver. Several studies have been done in this regard. A recent meta-analysis looked at 5 randomized controlled trials, comparing propofol and midazolam for EGD examination in patients with cirrhosis; it found similar safety for both drugs.[35] Psychomotor recovery was better in the propofol group compared with the midazolam group. NAAP was used in 3 of the 5 studies.

PSYCHOMOTOR RECOVERY

An important aspect of sedation in endoscopy that remains relatively understudied is after-procedure psychomotor recovery. The psychomotor effects of sedation include impaired physical and mental abilities. These impairments often require patients to take time off from work for the procedure and usually require a second person to accompany the patient to provide assistance until the effects of sedation are gone. The duration of impairment is mainly dependent on the type of agent used, the length of the procedure, and several other factors like patient age or BMI.[36,37]

Currently, most endoscopy units rely on the recovery of physiologic parameters, such as the Aldrete score (**Table 3**) and postanesthesia recovery score.[38] Some of the other tests available but less often used are the modified Gestalt test, reaction time test, driving simulator tests, and a Maddox wing test.[39] Willey and colleagues[37] were the first to address psychomotor recovery in patients undergoing endoscopy. The aims of their study were to determine the degree of psychomotor recovery after endoscopic sedation at the point of time when patients met discharge criteria and to identify a sensitive method for testing psychomotor recovery. All patients received midazolam and meperidine for sedation. By use of the Aldrete score at the time of discharge, the investigators found that those patients determined to be fit for

Table 3
Cardiopulmonary unplanned events

Category	Event	Definition
Cardiovascular	Hypotension Hypertension Dysrhythmia Cardiopulmonary arrest Myocardial infarction Cerebral vascular event	BP <90/50 or decrease in systolic pressure of 20% of baseline BP >190/30 or increase in systolic BP >20%
Pulmonary	Hypoxia Apnea/hypopnea Laryngospasm Bronchospasm Pneumonia Pneumonitis	SaO_2 <85%

Adapted from Romagnuolo J, Cotton PB, Eisen G, et al. Identifying and reporting risk factors for adverse events in endoscopy. Part 1: cardiopulmonary events. Gastrointest Endosc 2011;73:579–85.

discharge had achieved an average psychomotor recovery of 86.5% of baseline. They also found that the letter cancellation and multiple-choice reaction time tests had the highest sensitivity for detecting a depression in psychomotor function compared with baseline, with a mean recovery of 64% and 63%, respectively (P<.001).[37]

Propofol has a very rapid recovery time due to its favorable pharmacokinetic profile. Ulmer and colleagues[40] compared psychomotor testing in subjects randomized to receive midazolam/fentanyl or propofol administered by nurses under the supervision of a gastroenterologist. Psychometric testing was obtained at baseline and after recovery.[40] Subjects receiving propofol had improved psychomotor test results compared with subjects receiving midazolam/fentanyl. There are 2 studies that specifically measured time to return to driving after propofol-mediated sedation. Horiuchi and colleagues[38] prospectively studied the recovery of driving ability after upper-endoscopy procedure in 80 patients. The patients were randomly assigned to 2 groups: one that received an endoscopy unsedated and one that received an endoscopy with the standard single-bolus administration of propofol or midazolam. Driving skills such as tracking error, acceleration reaction time, and braking reaction time returned to baseline values within 60 minutes of propofol administration. In the midazolam group, significant driving errors were still evident at 120 minutes after drug administration.

In another study, Riphaus and colleagues[41] randomized 96 patients undergoing colonoscopy or upper endoscopy to midazolam/mepridine or propofol groups. In this study, a psychometric recovery using a number test and a driving simulator were used. The time to full recovery using a postanesthesia recovery score was significantly less in the propofol group. The number connection test values at 2 hours after recovery were the same for both sedation groups. Driving skills at 2 hours after propofol sedation were at baseline values, whereas in the conscious sedation group, lane deviations, reaction time, and speeding were significantly higher. A recent prospective study compared PADSS to clinical criteria for the determination of patient recovery before discharge. It clearly showed PADSS to be superior via allowing earlier discharge.[42] Concrete evidence is lacking as to which tools are best recommended for determining the safest time to discharge a patient. In the future, it is anticipated that there will be bedside computer models available to assess the recovery of psychomotor functions of a patient before discharge.

QUALITY IN ENDOSCOPY SEDATION

In recent years, there has been an increased focus on the quality of care surrounding procedures and health care in general. With reimbursements now tied to the quality of services provided, ASGE has developed various quality benchmarks for all endoscopic procedures. There are, however, no currently accepted quality measures for procedural sedation administration and monitoring.

The Iowa Satisfaction with Anesthesia Scale (ISAS) is an instrument that was developed to assess patient satisfaction with MAC.[43] The ISAS consists of 11 statements addressing a range of emotions and physical sensations, rated by patients (using a scale ranging from "disagree very much" to "agree very much"). The questionnaire is usually completed at the end of 24 hours after the procedure and has been validated in multiple settings.[43]

To address the same issue with moderate or conscious sedation, recently a large prospective study was done. This study by Leffler and colleagues[44] developed and validated a questionnaire to assess the quality of procedural sedation. The Procedural Sedation Assessment Survey (PROSAS) included a patient questionnaire after the procedure and the recording of sedation-related adverse events (SRAEs). SRAEs were recorded by a nurse during the procedure and were defined as follows:

1. Hospitalization because of an adverse event of sedation including aspiration
2. Use of narcotic or benzodiazepine reversal agents
3. Any episodes of oxygen desaturation less than 90% or leading to intervention
4. Any problematic changes in heart rate (heart rate <50 or >120) or BP (<90 or >160) during the procedure
5. Any hemodynamic or respiratory changes that interrupted the procedure

As part of their patient questionnaire, patients were asked about discomfort they experienced during the procedure, how much sedation would they prefer if they were to have the same procedure again, how much pain the patients had before the procedure, and how much pain they were experiencing after the procedure. All questions were answered on a scale of 0 to 10. The PROSAS is mainly based on patient input, although it does involve multiple stakeholders including clinicians. Also of note, PROSAS has incorporated adverse events as a reporting of quality in addition to patient experience, whereas the ISAS is only based on patient satisfaction. Although PROSAS does offer an opportunity to assess quality in conscious sedation, it still needs to be validated in other studies and across a wider population before it can be used as a metric for quality assessment.

At present, none of the endoscopy societies have clear-cut guidelines to measure quality for endoscopic sedation. ASGE in its 2015 guidelines on quality indicators for all endoscopic procedures did mention various indicators reflective of quality in endoscopic sedation.[45] In this they include patient monitoring during procedures, frequency of dosing medication and route of administration, use of reversal agents, and incomplete procedure or premature procedure termination as various quality indicators. Although these parameters are good, they are not comprehensive because it does not take into account patient satisfaction. Moreover, use of surrogate markers, such as need for reversal agents, probably is not the best indicator of quality measures. Perhaps as a first measure sedation, quality should be more rigorously implemented and studied. Consideration should be given to make it part of gastrointestinal quality improvement consortium, wherein it should include reporting of objective parameters as in patient vital signs during procedures, sedation-related complications, patient satisfaction after procedure. More studies are needed in this area to determine how to best measure patient satisfaction after procedure and also to test if surrogate markers like use of reversal agents do in turn reflect complications from sedation medications and can be used universally.

COMPLICATIONS

Procedural sedation-related complications remain one of the biggest challenges in current GIE. The definition of an unplanned cardiopulmonary event (CPE) is variable across the current literature. Because of this variable definition, reporting and recognizing CPE remain big challenges for practitioners and patients alike. The incidence of CPE reported in the literature varies from 1 in 170 to 1 in 10,000.[46,47] CPE remains one of the most commonly reported complications in GIE.

One of the biggest challenges in monitoring and reporting CPE complications is a lack of a universal standard definition. To address this challenge, an endoscopy workshop on adverse events was held in 2009. The main goal of the workshop was to supply a standard definition for sedation-related complications, and the minimum threshold of when the adverse events need to be documented and reported.[48,49] **Table 3** lists various CPEs along with standard, accepted criteria.

One of the important aspects for the prevention of sedation-related complications is careful hemodynamic monitoring. The ASGE and ASA Task Force on Analgesia by Non-Anesthesiologists recommend the use of continuous automated BP monitors during procedures. Early recognition of hypotension (a risk carried by the most commonly used sedation agents for GIE) will lead to early intervention efforts. Fisher and colleagues[50] evaluated 100 patients undergoing consecutive ERCP for CPE. The patients were divided into 2 groups based on their age: group 1 consisted of patients older than 65 years old, and group 2 consisted of patients younger than 65 years old. The study showed changes in electrocardiogram readings were noted in 24% of patients in group 1% and 9.3% in patients in group 2. Six patients showed elevated troponin levels after procedure in group 1, with 2 patients showing ST segments changes as well. The investigators concluded that a longer duration of procedure and congestive heart failure are risk factors for complications.

Transient mild hypoxemia is not uncommon and may be inconsequential. It is universally recommended to use pulse oximetry during endoscopic procedures, although there are no data to suggest that its use decreases the incidence of significant CPE. One meta-analysis found that the incidence of hypoxemia decreased by 1.5% to 3.0% with the use of pulse oximetry in the perioperative period, but this benefit did not translate to any mortality or morbidity benefits.[51] As of now, the ASGE and ASA recommend the continuous use of pulse oximetry during endoscopic procedures. The rarity of significant hypoxemia during procedures prompts a question regarding whether the use of capnography and extended respiratory activity can augment safety in GIE.

Recently, much interest has been generated regarding the use of capnography monitoring during procedures to improve hypoxemia detection rates. Capnography monitoring measures the carbon dioxide concentration throughout the respiratory cycle, which allows for real-time evaluation of a variety of respiratory factors, including respiratory depression, apnea, and hypercapnea.[52] The ASA updated the standards for basic anesthetic monitoring in 2010 (implemented in July 2011) that require capnography to be used for monitoring in all procedures using moderate sedation. The addition of capnography has been shown to decrease rates of hypoxemia with early detection of ventilation depression and allows for a more accurate titration of medications during procedures. Qadeer and colleagues[53] were the first to show a significant decrease in hypoxemia (defined as a SaO_2 <90% for ≥15 seconds) with open capnographic alarming during advanced endoscopic procedures. In the largest study to date, Beitz and colleagues[54] evaluated the use of capnography in 757 subjects undergoing a colonoscopy with propofol sedation. There was a significant reduction in the primary outcome of hypoxemia (defined as a decrease of >5% from baseline SaO_2 or <90% SaO_2 at any time during the procedure) in the open capnography alarm group.

No evidence existed until recently to suggest the benefit of capnography in GIE using moderate sedation. The authors' group, led by Mehta and colleagues,[55] studied the use of capnography in patients undergoing routine EGD and colonoscopy who are ASA class I and II. The study was a single-center, randomized, blinded, parallel group assignment trial that included the enrollment of separate EGD and colonoscopy groups. A total of 218 patients were enrolled for EGD, and 234 patients were enrolled undergoing colonoscopy. There was no significant difference in rates of hypoxemia between the EGD capnography blinded and open alarm groups. A total of 113 (or 54.1%) of all subjects had 1 episode of hypoxemia with a similar amount of events occurring in subjects randomized to the blinded (54.6%) and open alarm group (53.5%, $P = .87$). There was no significant difference in rates of hypoxemia between the capnography blinded and capnography open alarm groups. A total of 123 (or 53.2%) of all subjects had 1 episode of hypoxemia with a similar amount of events occurring in subjects randomized to the blinded (54.4%) and open alarm group (52.1%; $P = .73$). The investigators concluded that capnographic monitoring during routine EGD and colonoscopy with moderate sedation does not reduce the rates of hypoxemia in ASA class I and II patients.

The authors consider that capnography use is beneficial in cases of long duration and complex procedures, and in patients with an ASA class III or higher, or for patients with significant comorbidities. In patients with ASA class II or lower undergoing routine EGD and colonoscopy, the use of capnography may not be of additional advantage.

SUMMARY

Endoscopic sedation has evolved substantially over the past decade. Patient safety and comfort remain the center of focus. Even though a formal curriculum has been developed, there has not been, to the authors' knowledge, a competency-based sedation training program that has been implemented for endoscopic procedural sedation.

REFERENCES

1. Standards of Practice Committee of the American Society for Gastrointestinal Endoscopy, Lichtenstein DR, Jagannath S, et al. Sedation and anesthesia in GI endoscopy. Gastrointest Endosc 2008;68:815–26.
2. Hsieh YH, Chou AL, Lai YY, et al. Propofol alone versus propofol in combination with meperidine for sedation during colonoscopy. J Clin Gastroenterol 2009;43:753–7.
3. Patel S, Vargo JJ, Khandwala F, et al. Deep sedation occurs frequently during elective endoscopy with meperidine and midazolam. Am J Gastroenterol 2005; 100:2689–95.
4. American Association for Study of Liver Diseases, American College of Gastroenterology, American Gastroenterological Association Institute, et al. Multisociety sedation curriculum for gastrointestinal endoscopy. Gastrointest Endosc 2012; 76:e1–25.
5. DeMaria S Jr, Levine AI, Cohen LB. Human patient simulation and its role in endoscopic sedation training. Gastrointest Endosc Clin N Am 2008;18:801–13, x.

6. Trapani G, Altomare C, Liso G, et al. Propofol in anesthesia. Mechanism of action, structure-activity relationships, and drug delivery. Curr Med Chem 2000;7: 249–71.

7. Cohen LB, Wecsler JS, Gaetano JN, et al. Endoscopic sedation in the United States: results from a nationwide survey. Am J Gastroenterol 2006;101:967–74.

8. Stark RD, Binks SM, Dutka VN, et al. A review of the safety and tolerance of propofol ('Diprivan'). Postgrad Med J 1985;61(Suppl 3):152–6.

9. Short TG, Plummer JL, Chui PT. Hypnotic and anaesthetic interactions between midazolam, propofol and alfentanil. Br J Anaesth 1992;69:162–7.

10. McQuaid KR, Laine L. A systematic review and meta-analysis of randomized, controlled trials of moderate sedation for routine endoscopic procedures. Gastrointest Endosc 2008;67:910–23.

11. DeWitt J, LeBlanc J, McHenry L, et al. Endoscopic ultrasound-guided fine needle aspiration cytology of solid liver lesions: a large single-center experience. Am J Gastroenterol 2003;98:1976–81.

12. Riphaus A, Stergiou N, Wehrmann T. Sedation with propofol for routine ERCP in high-risk octogenarians: a randomized, controlled study. Am J Gastroenterol 2005;100:1957–63.

13. Dumonceau JM, Riphaus A, Schreiber F, et al. Non-anesthesiologist administration of propofol for gastrointestinal endoscopy: European Society of Gastrointestinal Endoscopy, European Society of Gastroenterology and Endoscopy Nurses and Associates Guideline—updated June 2015. Endoscopy 2015;47:1175–89.

14. Goudra BG, Singh PM, Gouda G, et al. Safety of non-anesthesia provider-administered propofol (NAAP) sedation in advanced gastrointestinal endoscopic procedures: comparative meta-analysis of pooled results. Dig Dis Sci 2015;60: 2612–27.

15. Rex DK, Deenadayalu VP, Eid E, et al. Endoscopist-directed administration of propofol: a worldwide safety experience. Gastroenterology 2009;137:1229–37 [quiz: 1518–9].

16. de Paulo GA, Martins FP, Macedo EP, et al. Sedation in gastrointestinal endoscopy: a prospective study comparing nonanesthesiologist-administered propofol and monitored anesthesia care. Endosc Int Open 2015;3:E7–13.

17. Ooi M, Thomson A. Morbidity and mortality of endoscopist-directed nurse-administered propofol sedation (EDNAPS) in a tertiary referral center. Endosc Int Open 2015;3:E393–7.

18. Virtanen R, Savola JM, Saano V, et al. Characterization of the selectivity, specificity and potency of medetomidine as an alpha 2-adrenoceptor agonist. Eur J Pharmacol 1988;150:9–14.

19. Candiotti KA, Bergese SD, Bokesch PM, et al. Monitored anesthesia care with dexmedetomidine: a prospective, randomized, double-blind, multicenter trial. Anesth Analg 2010;110:47–56.

20. Park HS, Kim KM, Joung KW, et al. Monitored anesthesia care with dexmedetomidine in transfemoral percutaneous trans-catheter aortic valve implantation: two cases report. Korean J Anesthesiol 2014;66:317–21.

21. Goudra BG, Singh PM. Propofol alternatives in gastrointestinal endoscopy anesthesia. Saudi J Anaesth 2014;8:540–5.

22. Lamperti M. Adult procedural sedation: an update. Curr Opin Anaesthesiol 2015; 28:662–7.

23. Bouvet L, Allaouchiche B, Duflo F, et al. Remifentanil is an effective alternative to propofol for patient-controlled analgesia during digestive endoscopic procedures. Can J Anaesth 2004;51:122–5.

24. Toklu S, Iyilikci L, Gonen C, et al. Comparison of etomidate-remifentanil and propofol-remifentanil sedation in patients scheduled for colonoscopy. Eur J Anaesthesiol 2009;26:370–6.
25. Miqdady MI, Hayajneh WA, Abdelhadi R, et al. Ketamine and midazolam sedation for pediatric gastrointestinal endoscopy in the Arab world. World J Gastroenterol 2011;17:3630–5.
26. Arora S. Combining ketamine and propofol ("ketofol") for emergency department procedural sedation and analgesia: a review. West J Emerg Med 2008;9:20–3.
27. Cohen LB, Cattau E, Goetsch A, et al. A randomized, double-blind, phase 3 study of fospropofol disodium for sedation during colonoscopy. J Clin Gastroenterol 2010;44:345–53.
28. Gan TJ, Berry BD, Ekman EF, et al. Safety evaluation of fospropofol for sedation during minor surgical procedures. J Clin Anesth 2010;22:260–7.
29. Pambianco DJ, Borkett KM, Riff DS, et al. A phase IIb study comparing the safety and efficacy of remimazolam and midazolam in patients undergoing colonoscopy. Gastrointest Endosc 2015;83:984–92.
30. ASGE Standards of Practice Committee, Chandrasekhara V, Early DS, et al. Modifications in endoscopic practice for the elderly. Gastrointest Endosc 2013; 78:1–7.
31. Mehta PP, Kochhar G, Kalra S, et al. Can a validated sleep apnea scoring system predict cardiopulmonary events using propofol sedation for routine EGD or colonoscopy? A prospective cohort study. Gastrointest Endosc 2014;79:436–44.
32. Young T, Finn L, Peppard PE, et al. Sleep disordered breathing and mortality: eighteen-year follow-up of the Wisconsin sleep cohort. Sleep 2008;31:1071–8.
33. Kaw R, Chung F, Pasupuleti V, et al. Meta-analysis of the association between obstructive sleep apnoea and postoperative outcome. Br J Anaesth 2012;109: 897–906.
34. Nagappa M, Liao P, Wong J, et al. Validation of the STOP-bang questionnaire as a screening tool for obstructive sleep apnea among different populations: a systematic review and meta-analysis. PLoS One 2015;10:e0143697.
35. Tsai HC, Lin YC, Ko CL, et al. Propofol versus midazolam for upper gastrointestinal endoscopy in cirrhotic patients: a meta-analysis of randomized controlled trials. PLoS One 2015;10:e0117585.
36. Dumonceau JM, Riphaus A, Aparicio JR, et al. European Society of Gastrointestinal Endoscopy, European Society of Gastroenterology and Endoscopy Nurses and Associates, and the European Society of Anaesthesiology Guideline: non-anaesthesiologist administration of propofol for GI endoscopy. Eur J Anaesthesiol 2010;27:1016–30.
37. Willey J, Vargo JJ, Connor JT, et al. Quantitative assessment of psychomotor recovery after sedation and analgesia for outpatient EGD. Gastrointest Endosc 2002;56:810–6.
38. Horiuchi A, Nakayama Y, Katsuyama Y, et al. Safety and driving ability following low-dose propofol sedation. Digestion 2008;78:190–4.
39. Horiuchi A, Graham DY. Special topics in procedural sedation: clinical challenges and psychomotor recovery. Gastrointest Endosc 2014;80:404–9.
40. Ulmer BJ, Hansen JJ, Overley CA, et al. Propofol versus midazolam/fentanyl for outpatient colonoscopy: administration by nurses supervised by endoscopists. Clin Gastroenterol Hepatol 2003;1:425–32.
41. Riphaus A, Gstettenbauer T, Frenz MB, et al. Quality of psychomotor recovery after propofol sedation for routine endoscopy: a randomized and controlled study. Endoscopy 2006;38:677–83.

42. Trevisani L, Cifala V, Gilli G, et al. Post-anaesthetic discharge scoring system to assess patient recovery and discharge after colonoscopy. World J Gastrointest Endosc 2013;5:502–7.
43. Dexter F, Aker J, Wright WA. Development of a measure of patient satisfaction with monitored anesthesia care: the Iowa Satisfaction with Anesthesia Scale. Anesthesiology 1997;87:865–73.
44. Leffler DA, Bukoye B, Sawhney M, et al. Development and validation of the procedural sedation assessment survey (PROSAS) for assessment of procedural sedation quality. Gastrointest Endosc 2015;81:194–203.e1.
45. Rizk MK, Sawhney MS, Cohen J, et al. Quality indicators common to all GI endoscopic procedures. Gastrointest Endosc 2015;81:3–16.
46. Silvis SE, Nebel O, Rogers G, et al. Endoscopic complications. Results of the 1974 American Society for Gastrointestinal Endoscopy Survey. JAMA 1976;235: 928–30.
47. Quine MA, Bell GD, McCloy RF, et al. Prospective audit of upper gastrointestinal endoscopy in two regions of England: safety, staffing, and sedation methods. Gut 1995;36:462–7.
48. Cotton PB, Eisen GM, Aabakken L, et al. A lexicon for endoscopic adverse events: report of an ASGE workshop. Gastrointest Endosc 2010;71:446–54.
49. Romagnuolo J, Cotton PB, Eisen G, et al. Identifying and reporting risk factors for adverse events in endoscopy. Part I: cardiopulmonary events. Gastrointest Endosc 2011;73:579–85.
50. Fisher L, Fisher A, Thomson A. Cardiopulmonary complications of ERCP in older patients. Gastrointest Endosc 2006;63:948–55.
51. Pedersen T, Nicholson A, Hovhannisyan K, et al. Pulse oximetry for perioperative monitoring. Cochrane Database Syst Rev 2014;(3):CD002013.
52. Vargo JJ 2nd. Sedation-related complications in gastrointestinal endoscopy. Gastrointest Endosc Clin N Am 2015;25:147–58.
53. Qadeer MA, Vargo JJ, Dumot JA, et al. Capnographic monitoring of respiratory activity improves safety of sedation for endoscopic cholangiopancreatography and ultrasonography. Gastroenterology 2009;136:1568–76 [quiz: 1819–20].
54. Beitz A, Riphaus A, Meining A, et al. Capnographic monitoring reduces the incidence of arterial oxygen desaturation and hypoxemia during propofol sedation for colonoscopy: a randomized, controlled study (ColoCap Study). Am J Gastroenterol 2012;107:1205–12.
55. Mehta P, Kochhar G, Albeldawi M, et al. Capnographic monitoring in routine EGD and colonoscopy with moderate sedation: a prospective, randomized, controlled trial. Am J Gastroenterol 2016;111:395–404.

Printed and bound by CPI Group (UK) Ltd, Croydon, CR0 4YY

08/05/2025

01864685-0001